Martial Arts for the Mature Athlete

A Guide to Injury Prevention and Treatment

John T. Hippen, MD

This book is dedicated to the memory of Scott Hoffman. He was a true friend and an honorable man. He was an inspiration in life and in death. He truly embodied the warrior spirit.

Acknowledgements

In the centuries since the Renaissance the modern world has often struggled with the balance between art and science. It is my hope that this book contains a little bit of both. Art and science can work together powerfully when they are both embraced and properly balanced. Medical science can and should help you in your study of the martial arts.

A special thanks to those who helped me in this work. First, thank you to my instructors and professors, both in medicine and in the martial arts. It is upon the shoulders of giants that I stand. I must confess a faith in higher power to have been so fortunate to be exposed to some of the great minds in medicine and in the martial arts world. It truly is an amazing time to be alive!

I would be remiss if I did not make particular mention of my instructor, Master Barry Barker and my wife, Doctor Rachelle Hippen. Without their help this book would not be possible.

Table of Contents

Introduction

As we age, the body changes. This is a natural, but not always desirable, process. I cannot even begin to count the number of times I've had patients look me in the eye and tell me, "Getting old is the pits!" or "Whatever you do, Doctor, don't get old!" The funny thing is the patients that tell me this usually aren't all that old. They are usually middle aged, and suffering the consequences of not having taken good care of themselves.

I have seen many people in their eighties and nineties who are still physically and mentally active. Most of them have in common one thing – they have *always* been active! The martial arts are one of those things that can bridge generations. It can teach the young some valuable lessons about life, it can impart everyone potentially life-saving skills, and it can keep the old going longer than they otherwise would.

With that said, it is not always easy being a mature athlete. It can be especially hard to start a new sport or to begin your martial arts journey when you are already in your forties or beyond. You cannot go back in time, though, and change the past. As the saying goes, "the best time to plant a tree is today."

I think you will find, however, that being mature is not always a disadvantage. When your knowledge and wisdom is combined with the right tools and a little perseverance, the possibilities are endless.

Section I: Key Elements to Success in the Martial Arts

Overview

So what is a mature athlete? Mature, in this context, simply means that you are not a child anymore. You are taking your training seriously and your body is fully-grown and developed. While there are certainly aspects here that would even apply to the child athlete or child martial artist there are other aspects that are unique to being an adult who is on his or her journey as an athlete and a martial artist.

There are plenty of children involved in the martial arts, and that is a great thing! Being an adult, however, you have certain strengths and certain limitations. In a world where there are far more children than adults in the martial arts this is sometimes overlooked. It is assumed that you too can touch your chin to your toes, do a back flip, a somersault, and then still come back tomorrow to do it all over again. For most adults, however, that is simply not the case.

This book will give you some tips on how to overcome some of those limitations and unrealistic expectations. So who or what exactly is an athlete? Let me make this simple. Everyone who is reading this book and ever has or will train in the martial arts is an athlete. I know some will balk at that statement, but if you get nothing more out of this book than that, I will have made a difference in your life.

In fact, I do not want you to keep reading until you can picture yourself as exactly that: an athlete. The reason for this is simple. If you expect to accomplish anything in your life with your mind and your body, then you need to train and prepare like an athlete. Even a brand new white belt is an athlete, and if he or she treats the body like an athlete would, what can be accomplished is astounding.

Let me talk for a moment about the counter argument to help you realize just how destructive it is. Perhaps you are thinking to yourself right now, "There is no way I'm an athlete." Or, "I'm just too old." Or worst of all, "I would never be able to do that." The next logical step is to have low expectations of yourself. After all, it is the safest way to go. "I'm just being a realist," you justify.

Realize right now that this can undermine everything that you can accomplish in the martial arts. This kind of attitude will frequently lead to you giving up prematurely. If you think this way, you won't train like an athlete, treat your body like an athlete, or eat like an athlete. Good athletes not only train for competition, but they train to win and they trains for life. They train to prevent injury and when they get injured, they train to overcome injury.

The fact that you are no longer as young as you used to be makes it all that more important that you train like an athlete. If you were a young healthy teenager you probably wouldn't need all that. Sure, it could still help, but it wouldn't be necessary. You could stay up late, eat poorly and still push through hours and hours of martial arts training without getting injured.

Now that you're not 13 anymore, you are going to need to take better care of yourself. The older you are, the more important it is that you approach life and the martial arts as an athlete. This one simple rule will benefit you tremendously, whether you are 19 or 90.

So let's get down to it. What are some of the key factors that are going to help you be more successful as you progress in your martial arts journey? Here are seven key elements that will help you along the way.

1. **Speed**

2. **Perseverance**

3. **Listening**

4. **Investing**

5. **Timing**

6. **Technique**

7. **Toolbox**

If you take the first letter from the seven key elements you will find that they spell the word **SPLITTT**. This is not coincidence. It is designed to help you learn, remember and incorporate these elements into your training. (It is a simple way to remember more information than you would otherwise retain and I bet if you asked your doctor, he or she had to do this about a million times to get through medical school.)

We will review each of the key elements briefly so you can see how it applies to you.

CHAPTER 1

Speed

Slow down! I still frequently teach martial arts classes despite my busy medical practice. I must admit, that sometimes I feel like a frustrated parent teaching his teenager how to drive. "Slow down" I yell in the vain hope that they will listen to me and remember to not drive so fast when I'm not watching.

This is one of the most important things that I can convey to you though. Speed is one of the biggest detriments to proper execution in the martial arts. Most good martial artists are NOT fast. Most fast martial artists are NOT good. Now there are exceptions. Bruce Lee is a popular example, but not everyone has that genetic gift.

Part of the problem is that a good martial artist who is also fast is very impressive. Everyone wants to move like him or her and so they try. Even worse, some realize that they don't know what they are doing, but think if they go fast enough no one will notice. I've got news for you – we notice!

I'll let you in on a secret. You know those very good and fast martial artists? You know the ones that I am talking about. They are the instructors and champions that you want to be like. Well, they did not start off fast. The best of the best learned to move with precision before they learned to move with speed.

Also, there are tremendous anatomical differences between children and adults. Their bodies are still developing. They are typically much more flexible, and as a general rule they can move through a range of motion in much less time. Because of their smaller frames they have a much smaller distance to move and much less mass to move as well. So slow down and let the kids go fast. Don't worry if that white belt next to you finished their form or kata well before you did.

Slowing down is one of the best things you can do for your body and your training. It will lead to more effective technique and reduce your risk of injury. An amazing thing happens when you move slowly and properly. With repetition you train the body and the mind. You are able to ingrain the movement neurologically. You make an imprint. Some call it muscle memory, but it is more than that. You are actually rewiring your body and your brain.

In time the speed will come, but when done properly that can take thousands of repetitions. Don't rush it though. If you do that you will still train your body, you will just train it incorrectly. If you speed up too early you will burn bad habits into your mind's memory banks that can take years to unlearn.

CHAPTER 2

Perseverance

Perseverance is a key element and it connects nicely with the idea of speed. Just as you need to slow down as you learn to perform each move correctly, you need to realize that you are not in a rush to get where you are going. If your first question when you enter a martial arts school is "How long will it take me to get a black belt?" or equivalent rank (black sash, instructors grade, etc.) then you probably need to take a step back and look at what your priorities are. If that is what is most important, there are much easier ways to "earn" rank these days. The only right way, if you are interested in developing lifelong skills, is through hard work. That will require a lot of sweat and maybe even little bit of blood and tears.

You probably get that already though. If you, as a mature athlete, are reading this book, then you already realize that you will not learn everything you need to know at once. It will take time and that is okay. You've already learned that most things in life that are worth doing are worth doing well, and that it takes time and experience to develop the skills that you set out to achieve. So take your time, be patient and don't give up!

I remember a black belt instructor who was asked how long it took for an average student to earn a black belt. He replied that *average* students do not become black belts. While that is certainly true, it is not usually the most talented or fastest learning students who do become black belts. It is those who keep going. I'll say it once more: DON'T GIVE UP!

CHAPTER 3

Listening

As newlyweds, my wife and I graduated from medical school in Washington, D.C. and moved across the country to start our respective internships. I can't tell you how excited my wife was to find out that as part of my pre-employment physical they would be testing my hearing. Because, she swore, I had to be going deaf at a young age. Shortly after we got married she had begun to notice that at times I would only pick up parts of conversations that we were having. To anyone that has been married before this may sound all too familiar!

Imagine her surprise when I returned home from my exam to report that I had passed the hearing test with flying colors. I was ecstatic! I was afraid that perhaps I really *was* losing my hearing. After all, as a newly minted medical student, I knew of all sorts of unusual conditions that could result in hearing loss. None of which I wanted, so I was elated by the news. She was absolutely dismayed. She could not figure out what was going on.

The interesting part is as we have been married longer, my "hearing", by my wife's own report has improved dramatically. I still have my moments, but by and large they have decreased. What happened? Did my hearing really improve? Of course not, I just learned to listen better. I had been suffering from the all too common condition known as "selective listening".

Not until I began practicing internal medicine and geriatrics did I realize how common this condition was. Certainly as we age there is greater hearing loss, and this is nothing to be made light of. I cannot tell you, though, how many times I have had spouses bring in their partners complaining of hearing loss only to find, sometimes after extensive testing, that there is absolutely nothing physically wrong.

Listening to your instructor is an invaluable part of being a student. Pay careful attention to what he or she is teaching you and implement it in your practice. Don't hesitate to ask questions at the appropriate time, but pay particular attention to the answers. If you ask the right questions, you will receive answers to your questions, and then some.

Perhaps even more importantly, though, I want you to learn to listen to your body. This is a skill that comes more naturally some than others, but I am convinced that it can be developed. Pain, aches, swelling, discomfort, and pressure are all signals that your body is sending you. You see, our bones, tendons, ligaments, and muscles aren't able to talk as our mouths do. They have a different way of communicating information to our brains. That information, when properly understood, can help you not only improve your technique, but also protect your body. It can help you avoid injury all together as well as recover from an injury when it has already been sustained.

So listen to your body! Learn to speak that language and understand what is being said. In time you will know when it is okay to push a little harder and when you need to ease back. Oh, and for you husbands out there, listen to your wives. Trust me, life will be a lot easier that way…

Chapter 4

Investing

This chapter is all about investing in yourself and your training and how to properly balance your portfolio. The investment analogy in the world of martial arts has many parallels to the world of financial investing. I am not an expert at investing money, but I do know a thing or two about investing your time into education, career, family, and last, but not least, the martial arts.

The world of financial investment can give you a better understanding, though, of how to invest your time in the martial arts. One of the first principles of financial investment is to start early. Another is to stay in it for the long haul. So if you are not already "investing" yourself in the martial arts but you want to, start now. If you already are doing this, keep going.

Part of what you need to know when you are investing in anything is what you want in return. For the martial arts, this could be self-defense skills, fitness, something in common with your children, improved confidence, or any number of other admirable goals. What you get back will be very different based on how you invest.

Let me give you an example. Robert has $1000 and wants to invest it to make some more money. An opportunity presents itself and he invests. Let's just say that he is fortunate, or smart, but he gets a fantastic return. His money doubles in just one year and he now has $2000. That is a lot of money to Robert and so he takes the money out and is quite happy, as any of us would be, with his $1000 profit.

Now let's say Sandy is in a very different situation. She can only afford to invest one dollar a day. She decides to start anyway because she has been told it is better to start early on investing even though she doesn't have anywhere near as much money as Robert. Unfortunately, she isn't as good at picking the perfect investment. Instead of getting a 100% return like Robert she only gets 10%.

So who is better off here? In our story, Robert just hangs on to that $2000 because he doesn't want to chance losing any of that money. Sandy, on the other hand just keeps putting in her one dollar a day. After just five years, Sandy will have more money than Robert. $2368 to be exact. In 10 years she will have over $6,000 – more than three times as much as Robert.

What does this have to do with martial arts? First, it doesn't matter what your starting point is. Sure it would be nice if you were already in shape or athletic. Perhaps you are naturally gifted and it comes easy to you, but perhaps you are not. Maybe you are a little bit more like Sandy. You aren't starting out with much and you can only invest a little bit at a time, but don't let that discourage you. Realize that there is no other place to start from then where you are already. Your persistence will pay dividends in time.

I still remember a friend I had that was training in Kenpo with me back in 1990 right around the time the movie *The Perfect Weapon* came out. He was taller, stronger, and definitely more athletic than I was. We had a competition at the school one day. We were each going to perform our forms or katas and the winner was going to take home one of the original movie posters.

I put everything I had into my performance, and by my standards at the time did a great job. I could not beat my friend though. He honestly did not train as hard as I did, but he was a natural. He pulled of his form like a seasoned pro. I finished second that day, but I didn't begrudge him his victory. He had earned it along with the poster to take home and put on his bedroom wall.

Shortly after that he stopped training. I would still see him from time to time, but he never did come back to train. A few years later I ran into him. He was doing other things in life and seemed happy. He was pleased with what he had learned while training. He was happy with the investment that he had made. Meanwhile I had moved into the advanced ranks and spent several days a week teaching classes at the school. My training had changed me physically and mentally. We both benefited from our training, but my return on investment was much greater than his.

It is also important to have proper balance in your investment. In the financial world they speak of this as diversifying your portfolio. There are two key ways to diversify your portfolio when it comes to the martial arts. The first is to balance your martial arts training with your personal, family, and work life. The second is to broaden your investment into more than one art. From plenty of personal experience with both I would like to give you some tips on how to do each successfully.

Whether you are running a family or a business, you have to be able to manage your money. The best way to do this is with a budget. Without a budget you just don't know where your money is going. Planning how you are going to spend your money makes a lot more sense than just hoping you have enough. When it comes to martial arts this principle also applies.

In the case of the martial arts, though, I'm not really talking about money. I'm talking about time. You need to have an idea of how much time you have in a day, a week, or a month and how you are going to invest it. The one difference here is that we all have the same amount of time in a given day. In those 24 hours, though, we all have different commitments. Some more and some less, but you need to make a conscious decision of how you are going to use that time.

Sure, you could just spend the day idly watching the world go by. You could surf the internet and play video games until you are hungry, then raid the fridge, and go back to the computer. The problem is, just like spending money without a budget, before you know it all your time is gone. I have friends who have done just that. They have spent their days having fun and doing whatever they felt like without any focus on where they are going and what they are doing. The days and even years go by faster and faster until you find that you really haven't done anything at all.

Regardless of how much time you have to budget for your training I want you to make a conscious decision. You should have an absolute minimum amount of time each week that you are going to dedicate to training. In this way, you ensure that you are at least making some progress. Obviously, the more time that you spend training, the easier it will be to progress.

A favorite quote of mine is from the Karate master Mas Oyama. He said, "Train more than you sleep." I must admit, though, that one of the reasons I loved the quote is that the first time I read it I was in my medical residency. At that time I would frequently go days at a time without sleeping. This made it very easy to train more than I slept!

In the real world most of us are going to sleep more than we train. We have jobs and families, communities and commitments. Make a conscious effort and a commitment right now to invest in your own life. The martial arts can be a good investment with excellent returns. Only you can decide, though, how much you can afford to invest.

I would encourage you to apply this to other aspects of your life. How much time are you dedicating to your family, your friends, your spouse, and your children? This should all be a part of your life budget too.

Cross Training

The next section I would like to discuss is how to properly diversify your martial arts portfolio. Most martial arts Masters that I know have trained in more than one art. There are exceptions, but by and large the best of the best have trained in more than one art or at least with more than one instructor. A great modern example is Dan Inosanto. He trained in Kenpo with Ed Parker before studying Kung Fu and Jeet Kune Do with Bruce Lee. He went on to train with Filipino stick fighting masters and the Machado brothers in Jiu-jitsu. He is one of the greatest living martial artists that ever lived.

Even the traditional martial arts masters that everyone looks to as having come from pure styles had multiple masters and arts. Gichin Funakoshi trained with multiple Karate masters before bringing Shotokan to Japan from Okinawa and thereby the rest of the world. Jigoro Kano trained with many of the best of his day before founding Judo and the Kodokan.

Now before you go running out to sign up for one week trial classes at every local dojo and school in your town think this through a little bit. The masters I mentioned above spent years training before they branched out. I have never met anyone who gained much of anything by training for a few days in a variety of styles. Even a few months of training is only enough to get a taste of what any particular art has to offer.

Now there certainly may be exceptions. I know of Jiu-jitsu schools that will have Judo classes to introduce students to takedowns that fit perfectly within the art they already practice. Your Muay Thai coach may have boxing class that he wants you to go to once a week after you have learned the basics. Your best guide is going to be your instructor. I don't ascribe to the rule that you must be a black belt or equivalent before branching out, but I do think it is a bad idea to sign up for 2 or 3 arts when you are just getting started. It is more likely to derail you or confuse you than it is to help you. If you're not sure, ask your teacher.

Chapter 5

Timing and Technique

Timing really is everything. Time applies to the martial arts in many ways some which we have already covered. First, what is the best time to start training? More often than not, the best time is right now! Don't hesitate.

Second, what is best amount of time to train? I would love to say 24 hours a day, but I know that isn't really true. You need to listen to your body to know what is the right amount of time for your body to progress while avoiding injury (more on that later). You also need to be able to look at your time budget and your other needs. Most of us aren't professional martial artists and so we also need to hold down a job in order to take care of ourselves, help our families, and still afford to train.

What I would really like to focus on, though, is timing and how that works with your proper technique. Any good martial artist can tell you how important this is. You can't learn it from a book, unfortunately. Just knowing about it, though, can help you be better attuned to it and apply it sooner. This goes back to one of my first points about speed and slowing your body down. One of the biggest reasons for this is it takes time for your opponent to react.

It is like playing pool and trying to take your next shot before the balls have even stopped moving. The most expert pool player waits for the shots to come to a stop, even though he knows exactly where they are going to stop. Think about that. There has to be time for him to respond and even if you are an expert when you are dealing with human beings, you don't know exactly what the reaction will be until it happens. So, wait! As you get better you will naturally speed up, but if you start off going as fast as you can you will never learn to do it right.

The next reason to slow down is to learn the rhythm of the art. I don't know of any martial art where this is more obvious than in Capoeira. When they spar or "play" it is actually a dance with music. There is a certain cadence and give and take that is expected while someone plays, either live or with a recording. It is the rhythmic music that guides the pace and rhythm of the exchange. This actually does exist in every other martial art, just to a lesser degree and without the music.

Think of boxing. Compared to Capoeira, it is decidedly different. Two heavyweight boxers going at it does not conjure the image of dancing. On the surface it is much more brutal and direct. Any good boxer will tell you, though, that rhythm is an essential part of the "sweet science". Trainers count out numbers and drills. They count out from the corners "Bob-weave-1-2. Bob-weave-1-2. 1-2-3. 1-2-3-4." There is a definite timing to it when a trained boxer practices his art. A good boxer knows how to break his own timing and his opponents so that he can direct the pace and rhythm of the exchange.

While I have trained in multiple arts I have spent more time in Kenpo than in any other. Kenpo has a decided rhythm to it. Some of the notes are short and others are long. Few instructors directly teach this rhythm though. That is not necessarily wrong, as it is more important to learn the basics first before overwhelming beginning students with the details of rhythm and timing. I know of too many brown and black belts, though, that haven't picked up on this yet. Once students memorize a sequence they blast through it as fast as they can.

A perfect example is Delayed Sword, which we call Delayed Hand. It is one of the first, if not *the* first technique that many Kenpo students learn. The reason it is called Delayed Sword or Hand is because students were moving too fast into the hand sword without proper timing or power into the move. For those who are not familiar with the technique, it is done with a right front hand grab or punch. The defense is to step back left with an inward block, followed by a lead leg kick, landing with a handsword strike. In the original technique, the front kick was not there. It was just block and chop. Having spoken to some of the senior Kenpoists who were there before the change say that what was happening was that most students were just blocking and chopping as fast as they could. As a result, the handsword had little power compared to what it could have. Mr. Parker as a result inserted the front kick in order to "delay" the handsword strike at the end.

Timing is a built-in part to every martial arts system of which I am aware of. Truthfully, it is a part of all sports, science, and medicine as well. Imagine a surgeon who wouldn't wait for a blood vessel to cauterize (stop bleeding) before moving on to the next part of surgery. He would quickly be out of practice as all his patients would be dead! Your best bet to figuring out the timing is to slow down and feel the timing. Experiment with different timing rhythms with your moves. Whether you practice Kenpo, Capoeira, Boxing, or Judo this will help you improve. Watch those more advanced students and instructors. Look for the breaks they put between their movements. There is often more than one "correct" timing so keep looking and listening and then feel the difference as you practice. Good musicians know that the most important part of music is not just the notes, but the space between those notes.

You might remember from our earlier mnemonic that there is actually a third T to know. That is your toolbox. This actually does not have to do with your technique toolbox it is about a literal toolbox. It is what you should have with you when you train. This part will make a lot more sense as you read the next section on *Injuries: Prevention and Treatment*. Let me give you an idea though before you head on to that section.

If you are lucky, your training location may have this already, but if not this is what you are going to need:

1. Athletic Tape
2. Ice Packs
3. Band-Aids or sterile coverings
4. Alcohol swabs or another topical antiseptic
5. An anti-inflammatory of choice (such as ibuprofen).

Additional items that aren't absolutely necessary but should be considered would include: compression wraps (ACE bandages), butterfly bandages, and petroleum jelly (Vaseline) or antibiotic ointment.

So we have talked a lot about some key elements that will lay you a great foundation for success in the martial arts and life. To sum it all up so far:

1. **Speed** – slow it down!
2. **Perseverance** – don't give up!
3. **Listening** – listen to your body.
4. **Investing** – think of the martial arts as an investment.
5. **Timing** – start training now!
6. **Technique** – slow it down and put some space between the notes.

7. **Toolbox** – be ready to train and for any injuries that may follow.

Remember, you are an athlete and need to train like one! You need to have the proper tools: mentally, physically and literally. Now that you have your mind ready and your bag packed let's talk about the body, those injuries, how to prevent them, and what to do when you encounter them…

Section II – Treatment of Common Injuries

Chapter 6

Using Your Toolbox

So now that you have your toolbox, what do you do with it? First and foremost, we hope we don't need it. The reality is though as any athlete will tell you – injuries happen. They aren't completely avoidable but they can be reduced. Once you are injured ignoring it won't usually help. This doesn't mean you have to go running to the doctor's office every time you bruise or sprain something. You will go broke just from the co-pays! When it is serious or not getting better you may need professional help, but I would like to guide you through some key steps in treating some of the more common injuries that you are likely to encounter along the way.

Let's talk first about how to prevent most injuries. Most people think if they just stay home and avoid any dangerous activities they will be fine. If you follow this line of thinking, before long, you will be a shut in. You will atrophy physically, your balance will worsen and your reactions will slow. I have seen more than a few people dedicated to this approach to life and help ruin their lives as a result. Before you know it, even walking becomes dangerous! Do not live your life in fear of getting injured. Realize that it will happen eventually, but that when it does, you will get better.

I'm not advocating that you deliberately put yourself in danger, but I have found that those who are absolutely obsessed with avoiding injury at all costs tend to be more prone to it in the long run. The above reasons are likely part of the reason why. In general, people who are more active do better! They feel better, are generally healthier and recover quicker from injuries.

I already mentioned earlier some of the ways to minimize injury. Slowing down and listening to your body are two great examples. Forcing yourself to go fast and ignoring the warning signals from your body are two sure fire ways to injure yourself. Another way to prevent injury is to realize that training is just that, training. It is not life or death. Whether you win or lose when you are training does not matter. You are there to learn not to win. This is one of the best signs of a mature martial artist. It is the person you want to be and it is definitely the person that you want to train with.

It is well known to most experience martial artists that the most dangerous person is not the master who has been doing this for years. He or she has great control and knows exactly how hard to push before letting go. He is able to pull that punch at just the last second to prevent a serious injury. The most dangerous is the brand new, gung ho white belt with the never say die attitude, a chip on his shoulder and something to proof. Please, do not be that guy!

One of the best ways to prevent injury is through training programs. Martial arts can certainly be a part of that program. There have been medical studies that have shown that strength and balance training along with stretching help to reduce the incidence of anterior cruciate ligament (ACL) tears in the knee. Similar studies have shown that wearing knee braces does not reduce the incidence of ACL tears.[1] There may be certain circumstances where braces, and compression in general, can be helpful, but your

---

[1] Prodromos CC, Han Y, Rogowski J, et al. A meta-analysis of the incidence of anterior cruciate ligament tears as a function of gender, sport, and a knee injury-reduction regimen. Arthroscopy 2007; 23:1320.

best bet is to train your body for the activity or sport you are participating in.

Some martial arts classes include this training as part of the program, but you don't need to be reliant on those alone to train your body and to prevent injury. Squats, calf raises and lunges in addition to running or cycling and stretching can help strengthen your body and prevent injuries to your body and especially your knees.

Now let's say that you've done everything right and you get injured anyway, what then? Let's talk for a moment about what you can do with some of those items mentioned above. For simple skin abrasions or cuts the appropriate use of antisepsis is generally self-explanatory, but in case it's not we will review it for a moment. First, clean the affected area. Soap and water, alcohol wipes, or hydrogen peroxide can all be used. Next, I recommend applying petroleum jelly (Vaseline) or antibiotic ointment and covering the area with clean bandage such as gauze with tape or a Band-Aid.

What about those painful sprains, muscle, bone and ligament injuries? You should be familiar with RICE if you are not already and I'm not talking about the fluffy white stuff that they serve with sushi. RICE stands for Rest, Ice, Compression, and Elevation. Rest means you minimize use of the injured area. If your ankle is sprained, don't walk on it. If your wrist is hurt, don't bend it. Ice can be applied to the area for 15 minutes up to every hour. Make sure there is something between the ice and your skin. Don't apply it directly or you can give yourself a case of frostbite! Compression means you wrap or brace the affected area. ACE wraps, neoprene braces, prefabricated splints, or lace up braces can all be used with good effect. In general, elevating the area can help reduce swelling especially when used in combination with compression.

For minor injuries, athletic tape is an invaluable part of the martial artist's toolbox. It works great for sprained fingers, wrists, ankles and toes and can be used elsewhere with success as well. If you've never taped yourself before find someone who has. They can give you tips and show you how to use it for best effect. There are entire books written on taping alone and I won't go into it in that kind of depth here.

The general principle is to stabilize the effected joint, but not to tape so tightly as to cut off circulation or make the area go numb. Usually wrapping the area at least two or three times is necessary. There are different taping patterns for different parts of the body that you will learn as you try this. This is something great to try on your more minor injuries so that when you have a more serious one you will already know how to do it. If you are not having success, seek out someone who has done this before who can give you some pointers. Having them show you once or twice how it's done will really jump start you in the right direction.

Another component of your toolbox that I recommend keeping on hand is an anti-inflammatory. The most common known ones, that I recommend, are ibuprofen (Advil, Motrin) or naproxen sodium (Aleve). These are not for everybody. If you have kidney disease, heart disease, or if you are allergic to any component you should avoid these medications unless your doctor tells you it is okay. Ibuprofen and naproxen work well for musculoskeletal injuries for two reasons. One, they are pain relievers. Two, they are anti-inflammatories as well, so they reduce swelling and inflammation which can help speed recovery from many common injuries. They are commonly called NSAIDs, which stands for non-steroidal anti-inflammatory drug.

This anti-inflammatory effect is best appreciated if they are taken close to the time of the original injury. That is why I recommend using it along with ice soon after you are first injured. For the most part, they should not be taken for a long period of time after the original injury. While I never recommend exceeding the recommended dosage, I tell most of my patients to "take it (the NSAID) like they mean it" for a few days up to a week. If they aren't getting better at that point, I generally want to know, but it is usually safer for them to take a higher dose for a few days then to take one or two tablets every day for the rest of their lives.

Chapter 7

Injuries to the Foot and Ankle

In order to be a good martial artist you need a solid foundation. With that in mind, we are going to work from the ground up going through some of the most common injuries martial artists and all athletes face followed by how to deal with them.

Toe Injuries

Toe injuries represent some of the most common injuries I have seen over the years. The good news is that they usually aren't serious. With that said, you must take good care of your feet. Repetitive injuries to the toes, or any body part for that matter, can lead to arthritis and chronic pain in later years.

Jammed, stubbed, sprained, or even broken toes are common. You typically recognize immediately when the injury happens that you did something wrong. The pain can be severe, especially at first, but these are injuries that don't have to stop you from training. Now, if you have a bone sticking out of your foot stop reading and go see a doctor. For the rest of you, you are going to want to get some good athletic tape and learn how to tape your toes and feet.

These toe injuries can take weeks and even months to heal, but if you tape them properly you can typically keep training. A great way to treat injured and even mildly broken toes is to buddy tape them. You will want to pick a toe next to the injured one and firmly tape the two together, wrapping completely around both toes several times. Wiggle the toes to make sure that one does not easily pull free. It should be more difficult to bend the injured toe, but it should not be numb. This may take a few tries to get it right if this is the first time you are attempting it. Don't worry, athletic tape is inexpensive.

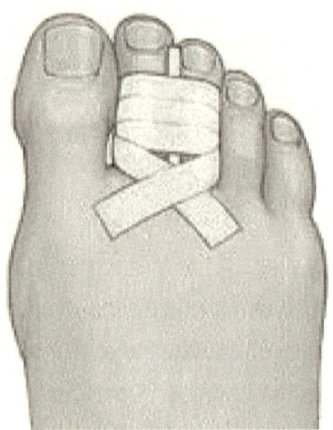

If the school where you train allows shoes, there is another option to buddy taping. As doctors, we will prescribe stiff post-operative walking shoes. They have a very stiff base that does not bend at all. You, also, can obtain such a shoe, or purchase a similar one that is very stiff as well. Typical training and running shoes are not adequate, as they are too flexible. If you want to wear a more comfortable athletic type shoe, you will need to buddy tape the toes.

Plantar Fasciitis

This is a common and painful injury for martial artists. You can recognize that you have Plantar Fasciitis by pain in the bottom part of the foot when walking. It is typically worse in the morning. The pain is usually in either the heel or the arch of the foot. This happens because the connective tissue that stretches from the heel to the ball of the foot actually slowly tears under pressure.

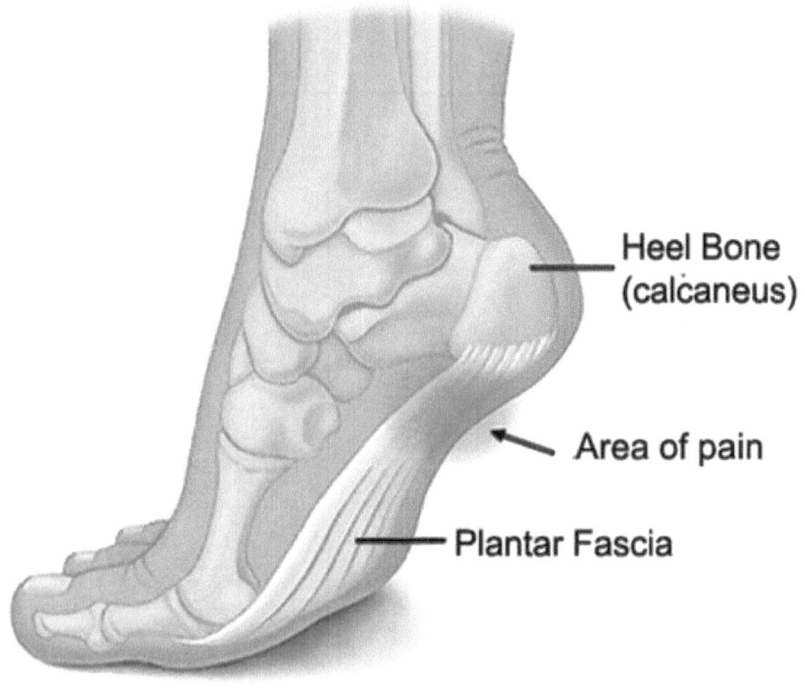

Heel Bone
(calcaneus)

Area of pain

Plantar Fascia

Whenever you are able to, wearing comfortable shoes with orthotics or arch supports can help expedite healing. If you must train barefoot, please tape your foot. Typically, you will need to tape lengthwise first along both sides of the foot and then wrap the mid-foot several times.

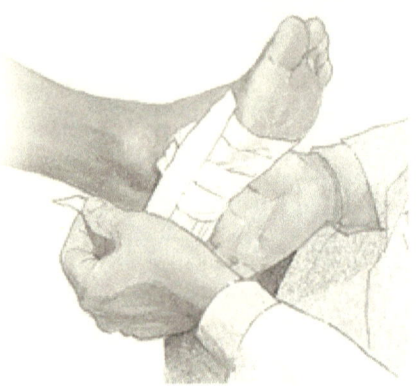

   In addition to orthotics and taping, massaging the affected area can also help speed recovery. A favorite exercise of many sufferers of plantar fasciitis is to roll a tennis ball back and forth under the foot a few times each day.

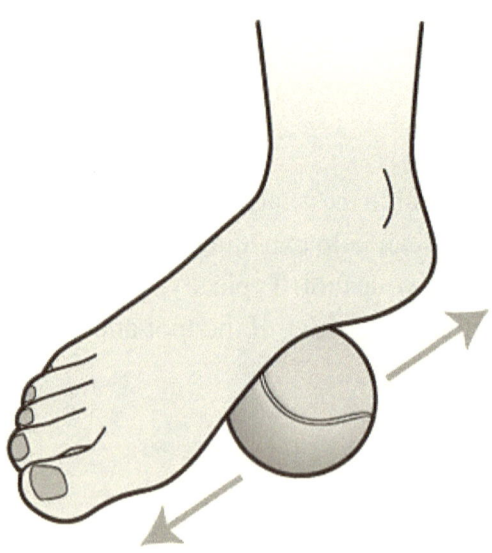

Strengthening and stretching the area over time can be very effective at easing the pain and preventing recurrence. I strongly recommend the following.

> Find stairs with a sturdy rail on which you can balance. While holding onto the rail, step onto the stairs with only your toes. Let your heels drop down as you stretch the foot and the calf. Hold that for a count of ten seconds. Then raise up onto the balls of your feet and hold that for ten more seconds. Repeat for a total of ten sets. Ideally, this should be done twice per day. This works best with shoes on as it minimizes the risk of overdoing it or injuring the foot.

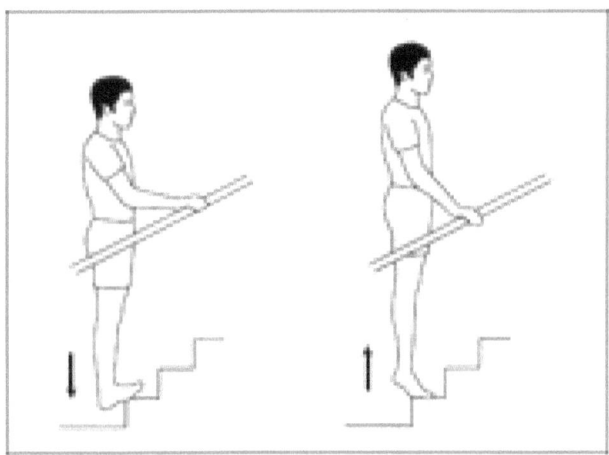

I would like to make a brief note about orthotics. Not everyone necessarily needs them, but if you have plantar fasciitis you likely do. The key is finding something comfortable that helps support the heel and the arch. You don't need to spend hundreds of dollars to get something custom-made. For most people, simple over-the-counter arch supports are sufficient. Studies have shown that inexpensive silicone heel cups that cost less than $10 work well and have similar results to arch supports costing much more.

Ankle Injuries

Ankles take a lot of abuse in many sports, and the martial arts are no exception. Unfortunately, if you have a badly injured ankle, rest is crucial to the healing process. While taping may help, if you are still having pain, you will be better-off staying off the ankle until it is healed. Ankles can be tricky for even the most experienced physicians to properly diagnose. Without imaging, such as X-rays, it is difficult to know if an ankle is just sprained, or if it is more seriously injured. If you are having persistent pain, tenderness, or trouble bearing weight, be safe and get an X-ray.

Rest, ice, compression and elevation (commonly known by the acronym RICE) are crucial to rehabilitating an injured ankle. If it is a sprain, RICE is likely all you will need to recover. If it is broken, however, you will likely need a cast to prevent further damage to the joint. Ignoring an ankle fracture is a recipe for disaster and may make surgery necessary, thus prolonging your recovery by months.

Some people are especially prone to ankle sprains because of their gait or the laxity of ligaments in their ankle, which causes them to repeatedly twist their ankles with exercise. Targeted training of the foot and ankle can help reduce that risk. The martial arts are a great way to strengthen an ankle. Another great strengthening exercise is to trace the letters of the alphabet with your toes. You can alternate between upper and lower case for variety. For example, this can be a great exercise to do when you are traveling on a long plane flight and want to keep the circulation in your legs moving, in order to prevent blood clots (which can occur with prolonged periods of sitting).

Achilles Injuries

Achilles tendinitis is the most common Achilles injury that I see. It tends to be chronic pain in the back part of the foot, just above the heel. Often times, people with this chronic problem will develop a bump at the top of the heel on the back of the foot. Achilles tendinitis tends to get worse with activity.

The first thing I recommend to treat it is a simple heel lift in your shoes. This will help when either walking or running. Second, you need to stretch your calf. If you can lengthen the muscle that attaches to the tendon, you will decrease the amount of strain on the tendon that occurs with activity. Almost any stretch of the calf can help. I would suggest starting with placing one foot behind the other as you lean into a wall. Be careful to keep the rear heel flat on the ground. This is a simple, yet surprisingly effective stretch that can be performed almost anywhere.

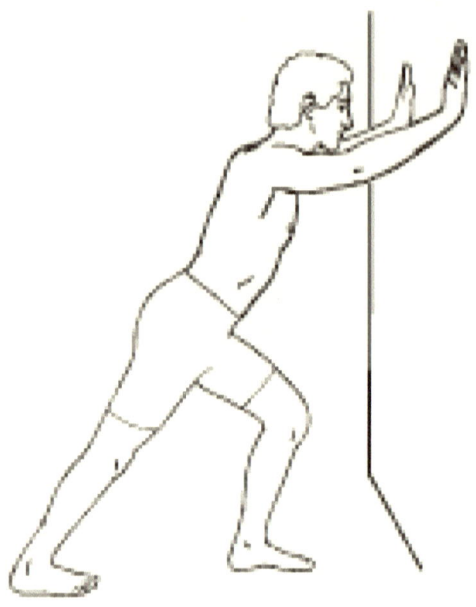

Achilles tendon rupture is a less common, but much more serious injury. It is a sudden tearing of the Achilles tendon and often requires surgery and a long period of recovery. If you regularly stretch the Achilles tendon and gradually strengthen the lower body, you are much more likely to prevent this type of injury.

Chapter 8

Injuries to the Knee and Hip

The human knee is an incredible joint. The balance of strength, stability, and mobility allow athletes to push their bodies and knees to extreme levels of performance. Unfortunately, there is only so much that the knees can take. As professional athletes have pushed their performance to higher and higher levels, their knees can't always keep up. While most knee injuries are not serious, some of them can be devastating.

ACL Injuries

An anterior cruciate ligament (ACL) tear is one of the most devastating knee injuries. It can often require surgery, followed by many months of prolonged rehabilitation. Even then, the after-effects can still limit mobility and cause pain, swelling, and arthritis for years to come. This is why athletes, coaches, doctors, and athletic trainers all agree that preventing ACL tears is so crucial. Martial arts training can certainly be a part of the training to help strengthen, stretch, and protect the muscles, tendons, and ligaments of the lower body.

There are five key parts to exercise regimens designed to prevent knee injuries and ACL tears. They are: warm ups, strengthening, plyometrics, agility and stretching. The following program is similar to programs that have been designed and proven to prevent ACL injuries, but it has been adapted to work with those practicing martial arts. The exercises are usually self-explanatory, but further information can be found at the Santa Monica Sports Medicine Foundation website at smsmf.org.

1.   Warm Up

a. Jogging

b. Sideways run or jumping jacks

c. Backward run

2. Strengthening

a. Walking lunges

b. Isometric/slow kicks

c. Single leg squats

3. Plyometrics

a. Jump squats

b. Jump switch front kicks

c. Jump switch back/rear kicks

d. Side to side jump side kicks

4. Agility

a. Sprints

b. Side sprints

c. High knee sprints

5. Cool down

a. Calf stretch

b. Hamstring stretch

c. Quadriceps stretch

d. Inner thigh/groin stretch

Knee Sprains

If you think you have an ACL tear, it is important to seek care from a healthcare professional. If you do, indeed, have a torn ACL, you will also need to see a specialist. Thankfully, most knee injuries are much less severe. A typical knee sprain is much more common, though, it can certainly put a damper on your martial arts training. The best treatment for a knee sprain is RICE (rest, ice, compression, and elevation) which I mentioned earlier. It is worth reviewing here in more detail since it applies particularly-well to knee injuries.

First, rest the knee. You should stop running or exercising if at all possible (i.e. if you are not being chased by a bear). If you have a more severe sprain, as indicated by pain simply with walking, then you may want to use crutches for some time. Second, you should also ice the affected joint several times per day. At least 15 minutes of icing is typically best, but you do not want to exceed 20 minutes. You should place a cloth or sheet between your joint and the ice so that you do not burn the skin (frostbite). Third, compression on the knee can be best performed using an elastic bandage (ACE) or a pre-fabricated knee sleeve. If you have a more severe sprain or a possible ligament tear, you may want to use a brace designed to immobilize the knee and completely prevent it from bending. Finally, elevate the affected joint. Ideally, the joint should be elevated above the level of your heart until the swelling goes down. One of the keys to healing the knee, or any joint for that matter, is to start the RICE treatment strategy as soon as possible.

Patellofemoral Syndrome

Patellofemoral syndrome is the most common cause of knee pain that I see in athletes, both young and old. It is a result of the patella (knee cap) not tracking straight on the groove at the end of the femur (thigh bone). It causes knee pain, usually after activity, though the knee can also become very stiff after sitting for a prolonged period of time. This has led to it being called "movie theater knee." This condition also leads to pain when going up and down stairs. Usually, but not always, the pain is worse going down the stairs as opposed to up.

In a normal, healthy knee, the patella sits right in the groove of the femur. This can be easily seen in a knee X-ray. Shown below is a normal knee X-ray taken from above the knee:

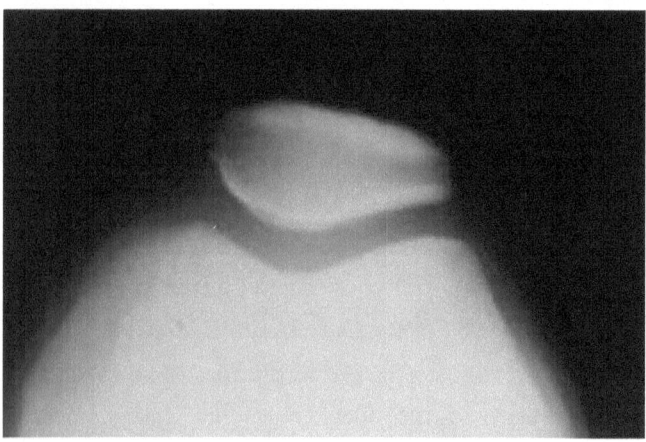

You can see the patella (the bone on top) sitting in the groove of the femur below it. In the next picture, you will see the patella pulled off to the side so it is not sitting in the groove any more. Picture it as two puzzle pieces that are not quite lined-up properly.

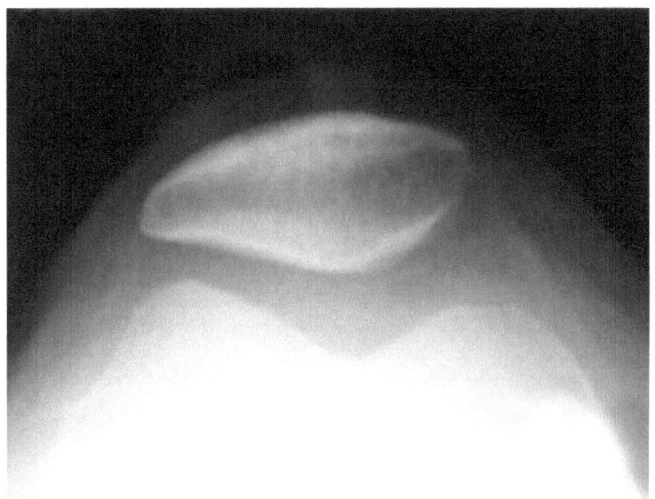

This results in pain and stiffness. Repeated bending of the knee will tend to increase the pain, while leaving the knee in a bent or flexed position for a long period of time will tend to result in increased stiffness.

The good news is that patellofemoral syndrome can most often be treated without surgery or medication. If the pain is severe, an anti-inflammatory medication (NSAID), such as Ibuprofen, may be beneficial in the short-term, but it is *not* a good long-term solution. The best answer is to strengthen the quadriceps (thigh muscles) to help the patella to start tracking straight and to get it to sit back in the groove again. We could subtitle this section: *How the Patella Got Its Groove Back*!

Almost all quadriceps-strengthening exercises are going to help to some degree. I generally recommend straight leg raises. To perform these, lie flat on your back with your legs straight and your toes pointing out at a 45 degree angle. Keeping the knee straight, raise one leg 18-24 inches off the ground and hold it for a count of 10 seconds. Bring that leg to the ground and repeat using the other leg. I generally recommend performing 10 repetitions with each leg twice daily. Although it can take weeks to see real improvement, it really does work. Surgery is *rarely* needed for this condition. If you are having trouble getting better on your own, an experienced physical therapist can be a tremendous help.

You can supplement with other leg-strengthening exercises, such as body-weight squats and lunges. You should avoid leg extensions however. The repeated bending of the knee, especially under a load, can exacerbate the pain.

Hip Injuries

Iliotibial Band Syndrome

Iliotibial (IT) band syndrome is a common cause of both knee and hip pain. The IT band is a connective tissue that connects the ilium in the pelvis to the tibia just below the knee. IT band syndrome can cause tightness and pain anywhere from the hip to just below the knee, but the most common places to have pain are the side of the hip joint and the outer side of the knee. It frequently results in a popping sensation in the hip. It can be frightening when it happens, but it is generally not serious. Stretching the IT band can help minimize the pain and stop the popping.

While RICE can help some as well, stretching the IT band is really the ideal treatment. One of the best ways to do this is to bend forward at the waist while keeping your legs straight and trying to touch your toes. Crossing one leg over the other will increase the amount of stretch on the IT band and stretch the hamstrings a little bit less. I recommend stretching for about one minute on each side and then repeating again. From that position, you can lean into the affected hip and support yourself on a wall, desk or partner to get an even greater stretch of the IT band.

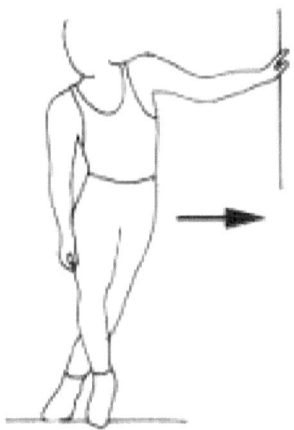

Trochanteric Bursitis

When the IT band is tight enough and continuously rubs on the outer part of the hip (the greater trochanter) in can result in a condition called trochanteric bursitis. Trauma to the area can also result in trochanteric bursitis. A bursa is a lubricating sack of fluid that surrounds the joint. When it gets injured or inflamed, we call it bursitis. In order to help this heal, I would recommend you follow the RICE treatment pattern. If it is still not getting better, you may benefit from physical therapy or a localized injection directly into the bursa. The stretches above may also help, and topical anti-inflammatory treatment, such as ice or trolamine salicylate (sold under the brand name Aspercreme) are also frequently beneficial.

If the hip pain is chronic or worsening, further evaluation may be warranted in order to rule out a more serious condition. Stress fractures, arthritis, and impingement are potentially serious conditions that can also affect the hip joint. RICE, stretching, and NSAIDs are generally effective; however, when they aren't, you may need to seek professional medical advice.

Chapter 9

Injuries to the Hand and Wrist

The hand and wrist are possibly the most critical areas to protect during martial arts training. The hands, especially the fingers, suffer a lot of abuse during martial arts training. Not only are the hands and fingers crucial for routine daily activities, for many people, they are the key to their livelihoods due to their use in their jobs. Thus, prevention of hand and wrist injuries is critically important.

I would like to start by addressing the controversy over hand conditioning, which includes things like knuckle pushups, punching a makiwara board, and jamming your hands and fingers into sand and rocks. In general, I am against it. That is not to say that you can never do knuckle pushups or punch a makiwara board, but what I am saying is that you should not engage in hard core, old school "iron palm training." These activities have very little benefit in your daily training regimen. In addition, even if you do not suffer any serious injuries now, you will likely have arthritic pain as you get older.

It is also important to realize that most injuries actually occur during sparring, not competition. Whether you call it sparring, randori, kumite, or rolling, there is a definite risk of significant hand injury. In order to prevent injury, you need to appropriately protect your hands and fingers. If you box, proper hand wraps and boxing gloves are critical. And you must make sure that you know how to wrap your hands properly, so that the wraps can give you adequate protection.

If you practice mixed martial arts or karate and use open-finger gloves, be very cautious. Learning to keep the fist closed when not grabbing may save a finger. Taping the fingers, hands, and wrists can also be a very good idea if there is a higher level of contact, such as at a competition. If you practice judo or jiu-jitsu gloves are not worn, but learning to properly tape your fingers can be very helpful. If you have any doubts about the need for taping, next time you watch a judo or jiu-jitsu tournament, take notice of how many of the black belt level competitors have their fingers taped.

Broken and Sprained Fingers

Sprained, jammed and hyperextended fingers can and *will* happen frequently, and taping the fingers can help significantly. You can either buddy tape the fingers for more support (see Chapter 7 for more information on buddy taping), or tape each finger. If the sprain is more severe (or the finger is broken) you will want to place the finger in a split. Cushioned aluminum finger splints are available at most pharmacies.

If the finger is fractured, good alignment is essential to proper healing, and can be verified by X-rays ordered by your physician. It is crucial to seek medical attention immediately, if you suspect a fracture, as the bones must be aligned properly before they start to heal. This will ensure that once the bone is healed, you will not lose any function. Particularly serious fractures can sometimes require surgery to repair them.

Mallet finger is a common name for a finger injury that causes damage or a tear of the ligament. This leads to an inability to straighten the finger. In this case, if the finger is not properly splinted, you may end up with permanent limitations in your ability to straighten the finger. Special splints are needed to treat mallet finger, and medical attention should always be sought when a finger injury leads to the inability to straighten the finger.

Another common injury is called an avulsion fracture. This occurs when the finger trauma causes the ligament to pull so hard at the attachment point on the bone that it actually breaks off a piece of the bone. This too, is treated with splinting.

Boxer's Fracture

A Boxer's fracture is a through the bones that form the knuckles of the ring finger and/or pinky finger (called the metacarpal bones). This type of fracture occurs when a hard object (such as a wall) is struck with the closed fist. If you do suspect a Boxer's fracture, you should get X-rays immediately. If confirmed, this type of fracture will require casting, and sometimes surgical repair, leading to months of recovery time before a return to training.

For this reason, it is critically important to learn to punch correctly so that you can prevent this type of fracture. Punching with the first two knuckles (as opposed to the knuckles of the ring and pinky fingers), is crucial, as these are stronger and thicker than the other bones, and are thus less likely to break after a hard impact. The last two knuckles, in contrast, can break fairly easily with even a moderately forceful punch. So, punch properly and don't break your hand!

Wrist Injuries

Wrist injuries can be very frustrating. One of the most common complaints I get from martial artists and other active people when they injure their wrists is that they cannot perform pushups. Unfortunately, there is no good way around this. You need to avoid the typical push up position until the wrist heals. You will just have to be creative and find other ways to work out!

RICE, along with bracing and taping, can help sprained wrists to heal and allow you to continue with your training. You want to make sure not to tape the wrist so tightly that you compress the artery in the wrist (called the radial artery) and cause the hand to go numb. Gentle range of motion exercises such as rolling the wrist clockwise and counter-clockwise can help improve range of motion. Gentle flexor and extensor stretches (see figures 2 and 3 below) can also help.

Wrist fractures on the other hand, must be taken seriously. Because the bones are often not aligned properly, they frequently require surgery. Arthritic pain and loss of range of motion are common consequences of wrist fractures that are not properly and promptly treated.

Carpal Tunnel Syndrome

While carpal tunnel syndrome (CTS) is not a condition that is typically the direct result of practicing the martial arts, it is very common in the general population, and thus is seen in many martial artists as well. It occurs as a result of pressure in the wrist on the median nerve as it passes through a ring of fibrous connective tissue at the wrist joint through which pass the nerves and blood vessels from the arm into the hand, called the carpal tunnel. The primary symptom is a numb sensation, with or without pain and weakness, in the hand and fingers. Many people with CTS also experience a loss of grip strength. CTS occurs most commonly as the result of typing, computer work, and repetitive hand use. Since many of our jobs include this type of work, it is important to be aware of it. Because CTS can cause numbness and weakness in the hand, it will definitely affect your ability to practice the martial arts. While carpal tunnel release surgery is often successful, it carries with it a long period of recovery, and is usually avoidable if you treat the condition initially with more conservative measures.

The first step in the treatment of CTS is to determine what activity is causing the symptoms. What are you doing that is putting pressure on the carpal tunnel and consequently the median nerve? Pay particular attention to computer, keyboard, and mouse use, as well as any activity with the arms or hands that you do consistently and repetitively. In order to reduce the symptoms, you will need to modify or minimize those motions that are causing them. If you are resting your hands on a desk or keyboard as you type or use the mouse, this may be the cause.

Unless your symptoms are very mild, you will want to brace the wrist as well. Using a wrist cock-up brace (also known as a carpal tunnel brace) you can help protect the median nerve and speed healing. The most beneficial time to wear the brace is at night. Many of us naturally bend our wrists at night while we are sleeping, which results in a compressed median nerve. The wrist brace can prevent that from happening. If you are having significant daytime symptoms you may need to wear the brace during the day as well. In severe cases of carpal tunnel, you may need to wear the brace both day and night until the symptoms improve.

Stretches can also help improve function of the hand and minimize carpal tunnel symptoms. The prayer stretch, flexor stretch, and extensor stretch shown below are three great stretches to help your carpal tunnel syndrome heal.

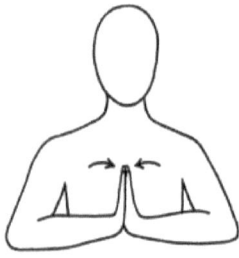

Figure 1 – Prayer stretch

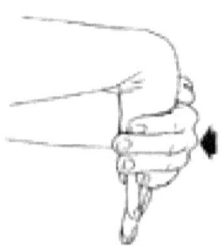

Figure 2 – Flexor Stretch

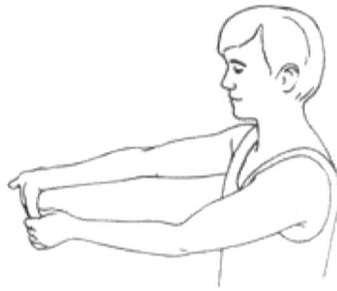

Figure 3 – Extensor Stretch

If stretching, along with a wrist brace, does not relieve your symptoms, you may want to discuss with your physician whether a Cortisone injection may be indicated. While this injection can be helpful in the short-term, the relief is often temporary, especially if you do not eliminate the inciting activity and continue with your stretching exercises. There are, however, some special circumstances, such as in pregnancy and the immediate post-partum period, where Cortisone injections, combined with wrist bracing and proper stretching, can lead to permanent relief of symptoms. If, after all of the above measures, you still have severe numbness, weakness, or pain, you may ultimately have to consider carpal tunnel release surgery.

Chapter 10

Injuries to the Elbow and Shoulder

Elbow and shoulder injuries are common for nearly all athletes, and martial artists are no exception. While I do see some blunt force injuries to the elbow, the most common causes of elbow pain are lateral and medial epicondylitis, more commonly known as tennis elbow and golfer's elbow, respectively.

Tennis and Golfer's Elbow

Tennis elbow occurs when the tendons rub on the outer part of the elbow (or epicondyle) and start to tear, leading to inflammation. The more you use the arm, the worse it gets. Rest and ice can help, but the challenge with that is how difficult it is to truly rest the elbow, given how much we use are arms in our daily routine activities. Tennis elbow can easily become a chronic condition unless you are able to stop the ongoing inflammation and damage to the tendons in the elbow.

While ice and NSAIDs can temporarily relieve the pain, ultimately you need to get the tendons to stop rubbing on the bony part of the elbow joint. One the best ways to do this is with a tennis elbow brace. The brace actually sits on the thickest part of the forearm just below the elbow. It applies pressure to the muscles and tendons. The muscles are still able to contract, but this stops the tendons from repeatedly rubbing back and forth over the joint. This brace usually needs to be worn twenty-four hours a day for at least six weeks in order for the tendons to fully heal.

The best strategy to prevent damage to the tendons in the elbow is to stretch the muscles in the forearm. By stretching, you take the tension out of the tendon and allow it to move about without grinding or catching on any part of the joint. Think of it as similar to loosening an overly-tight guitar string - if the string is too tight it is likely to wear thin, then fray, and eventually break. Once you start loosening it, you can start to notice a difference right away.

The best and simplest stretches for the forearm can be done using your opposite hand or a wall. With the arm extended out in front of you, first point your fingers down, with the arm fully bent at the wrist. Using a wall, or your opposite hand, gradually apply increasing pressure until you can feel the stretch in the forearm. Hold that for about one minute. Next, repeat the stretch with the fingers pointing up. Then, repeat the cycle again. Doing this once or twice a day will reduce the tension in the tendons and prevent further injury while they heal.

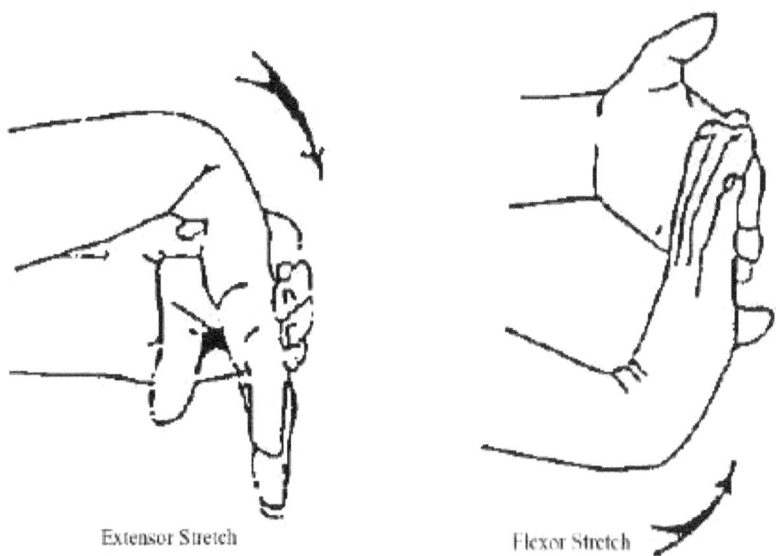

Extensor Stretch   Flexor Stretch

The cause of golfer's elbow is similar – tendons in the elbow begin to rub on the bony part of the elbow and slowly tear.

The difference in this case, however, is that the affected tendons are on the inner part of the elbow instead of the outer part seen in tennis elbow. The treatment for golfer's elbow is also almost identical to that of tennis elbow - bracing and stretching are still the best strategy.

If the stretches and bracing don't work, you can consider having your doctor perform a cortisone injection in the elbow. These often provide temporary relief, but they are not without risks. One of the main problems with the injections is that once the injection relieves the pain, people tend to stop wearing the brace and stop stretching, because the elbow feels so good. Then, once the effects of the injection wear off, if you have not kept up with the bracing and stretching, the pain returns. This leaves you back where you started.

Physical therapy can be a big help for those with chronic or recurrent symptoms from tennis elbow or golfer's elbow. Although still not used consistently in main-stream medicine, some physicians also treat tennis elbow and golfer's elbow with injections of platelet rich plasma (PRP), which can be helpful in some cases. There are also pain-relieving patches that some sufferers find helpful. Surgery is a last resort, and is usually only needed in the most severe cases when everything else has failed.

Olecranon Bursitis

Another cause of elbow pain is olecranon bursitis. In this condition, the outer surface of the elbow becomes inflamed and swollen. It can occur due to direct trauma to the area. Less commonly, hyperextension can injure the olecranon (part of the ulna, a forearm bone), and result in bursitis. The olecranon is the part of the ulna that connects to the humerus (upper arm bone). The bursa sits just outside the ulna.

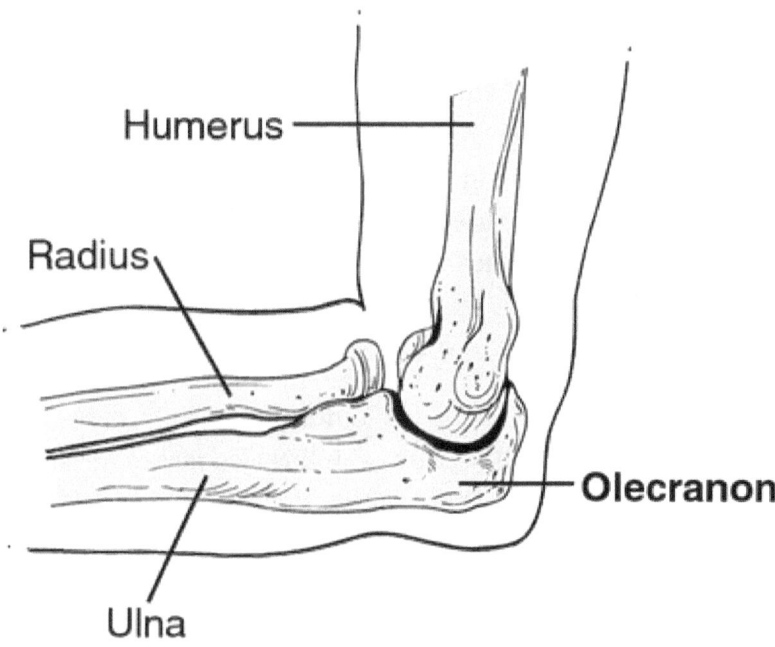

Humerus

Radius

Ulna

Olecranon

If the bursa is injured, it can result in pain and dramatic swelling. If the pain and swelling are mild, you should use the RICE method as discussed previously. If the swelling is considerable, you may want to see a physician, who can drain the fluid, thus relieving the pressure. Once the fluid is drained, it can be sent to the lab to test for the presence of infection. If you are unable to fully move the arm at the elbow joint after trauma to the area, I would recommend an X-ray to make sure that there is no underlying fracture. Bursitis causes pain and swelling, but in most cases, it shouldn't keep you from moving the arm. If you cannot move the arm, there is likely something else causing your symptoms.

Shoulder Pain

If you are a martial artist with shoulder pain, don't worry, you are in very good company. Most martial artists will have shoulder pain at some point in their lives. Chuck Norris made the Total Gym famous after he used the machine to rehabilitate his injured shoulder and then became their official spokesperson. If someone like Chuck Norris gets shoulder pain, surely the rest of us are not immune!

The shoulder is an incredible joint because it offers so much mobility and versatility. However, this also makes it less stable and puts it at higher risk for injury. Because so many working parts are needed to achieve this versatility, there are also numerous potential causes for a given case of shoulder pain. One of the most common causes of shoulder pain is tendinitis. This, by definition, is inflammation of the tendons in the shoulder joint. It can affect both the rotator cuff tendons as well as the biceps muscle tendons that attach the muscle in the upper arm to the shoulder. Two other common shoulder injuries are shoulder dislocation and tears of the lining of the shoulder capsule (called the labrum).

Rotator Cuff Injuries

The rotator cuff is actually made up of a group of muscles and tendons that all work together to move and rotate the shoulder. As you get older, unfortunately, they become thinner and more prone to tears. After the age of 45, your risk of a rotator cuff tear is significantly higher. However, even younger athletes frequently injure the rotator cuff tendons due to repetitive and rapid, powerful motions. If you have a rotator cuff tear, you may need to have surgery, though this is not a foregone conclusion. All rotator cuff tears do not necessarily need surgery, and, in fact, many can resolve completely with the proper treatment regimen. This is a situation, though, where you will likely need to see a specialist to discuss your treatment options.

Although rotator cuff tears can be very painful and devastating injuries, at all ages, tendinitis of the shoulder is still much more common than a tear. Although tendonitis can still cause significant pain, the prognosis is generally much better than for tears.

The hallmark feature of tendinitis is pain with specific types of motion of the arm. This pain eventually causes you to avoid certain activities with your shoulder, which can lead to a gradual stiffening of the joint. Pain when reaching up, across, or back behind you are some of the most common complaints in rotator cuff tendonitis. Since there are four rotator cuff muscles surrounding the shoulder, pain can be in the front, back, or side of the shoulder.

Heavy overhead lifting can further damage the rotator cuff muscles, and should be avoided while the shoulder is healing. Ice can be very beneficial, as can topical and oral anti-inflammatories (NSAIDs). Using a shoulder sling is generally not recommended because, while it can help relieve the shoulder pain, its use for more than a few days can result in a stiffening of the shoulder and a loss of the normal range of motion (commonly called frozen shoulder).

There are a few key exercises that can help with rotator cuff tendinitis. The first is called the wall crawl. Use your fingers to "walk" up a wall as far as you can without pain, then repeat. It is important to use your fingers (not your shoulder) to support the weight of your arm while doing this exercise. This exercise can help improve the range of motion in the arm and also help prevent frozen shoulder.

A second exercise to help with rotator cuff tendonitis is called the pendulum exercise. While holding a very light weight object in your hand (such as a water bottle or can of soup), bend at the waist 90 degrees, and then swing the arm back and forth. You can also make a circular motion with the arm, moving in a clockwise direction for 30 seconds, followed by a counter-clockwise direction. Keep going for about 2 minutes and repeat multiple times.

If these exercises are not helping, your pain is getting worse, or you are over the age of 45 you may wish to see your physician. Physical therapy can again be very helpful in restoring the strength and the range of motion of the shoulder. Injections can also be very helpful for shoulder injuries that are not improving on their own.

Biceps Tendinitis

Biceps tendinitis feels very similar to rotator cuff tendinitis, so much so that it can sometimes it can be tricky to tell the two apart. Fortunately, the same treatment that helps the rotator cuff can help the biceps tendon as well.

In biceps tendinitis, the front part of the shoulder tends to be the most painful. It causes pain when lifting the arm in front of the body, as well as with flexing the elbow against resistance (the same motion used during dumbbell or barbell curls). In contrast, with rotator cuff tendinitis, it is usually overhead lifting that is the most painful.

RICE tends to be the best approach once again for treating this ailment. The stretches described earlier for rotator cuff tendinitis can be quite helpful in biceps tendonitis as well. One of the most important factors in healing the biceps tendon is determining exactly what activity that you are performing is causing the injury, so that you can start avoiding it.

As the father of a young child, I have witnessed first-hand the pain that can result from certain repetitive motions of the shoulder. As he has continued to grow older (and heavier), the pain in my shoulder also began to grow more intense and more frequent. I have noticed, however, that simply switching from carrying him with my right arm to my left arm (thus eliminating the inciting activity), has helped to reduce the pain considerably in that right shoulder. I have come to realize that, as long as I frequently rotate which arm I am using, I can avoid the pain normally associated with these types of repetitive arm motions. My story is not unusual. Many men and women will tell you similar stories of pain in the shoulders along with pain in the elbows, wrists and hands that started after they became parents. This illustrates an important lesson - as a martial artist it is important to realize that sometimes it is not always the hard training that you do once or twice a day that results injuries, but instead is the repetitive motions that you do hundreds of times a day, either at home or at work, that cause the most pain.

Shoulder Dislocations

Many martial arts techniques are designed to lock or dislocate the opponent's shoulder. With proper training and good training partners, hopefully you never suffer this injury. While training, use caution when performing these shoulder locks on your training partners, and be certain to stop when they indicate that they have had enough. If you find yourself caught in one of these locks, or any lock for that matter, while sparring, do not let pride keep you from submitting or tapping your partner so that he or she knows stop. It is better to lose the match, learn a lesson, and preserve your shoulder joint than to have your shoulder dislocated.

If you do suffer a shoulder dislocation it is important that you have it set properly. There are "battlefield" techniques for setting a shoulder, but I would not recommend that you try them unless you have had professional training. If you do not understand the anatomy of the shoulder joint, you are more likely to do more damage than good if you try to reduce the dislocation yourself. You will be much better off in a physician's office, with pain medication and X-rays, than you would be with your training partner standing on your chest and trying to pull your arm back into the socket, not realizing that he or she may very well be pulling the wrong direction!

Once the shoulder is set by a professional, follow the RICE principles discussed earlier. Rest is crucial, as shoulders will take time to heal and you don't want to reinjure yourself by coming back to training too soon. Recurrent shoulder dislocations can have devastating long-term consequences, so avoiding that at all costs is key. Be patient!

Labrum Tears

The labrum is a rigid type of cartilage found in the shoulder joint. It is located around the socket where the upper arm (humerus) attaches at the shoulder. The humerus bone forms a "ball" shape at the end (called the head of the humerus), and the labrum helps to keep that ball inside the shoulder "socket." In addition, the biceps tendon that was discussed earlier, attaches to the labrum at the shoulder joint. One of the dangers of dislocating the shoulder is that you can also injure or tear the labrum in the process. This results in recurrent pain and makes it much easier to dislocate your shoulder in the future. This can result in a clicking sensation in the shoulder as the head of the humerus rubs against the torn piece of the labrum.

The initial treatment for a labral tear would still be RICE, and it may also benefit from an injection or physical therapy. However, if it is anything more than a minor tear, you will likely need surgery to repair it. This is another situation where consulting a sports medicine or orthopedic specialist will be crucial.

Chapter 11

Injuries to the Chest and Back

Chest Pain

Very few things frighten people more than chest pain. My goal here is not to discuss the diagnosis and treatment of heart disease. Suffice it to say that a healthy lifestyle, including proper diet and physical activity (such as the martial arts) can reduce your risk of heart disease. If you are experiencing chest pain with exertion, though, you should seek medical advice immediately. Other common symptoms of heart-related conditions include shoulder pain, jaw pain, profuse sweating, and nausea.

The most common athletic injuries involving the chest that I would like to discuss are rib injuries (fractures and sprains) and chest wall contusions (bruises). Unfortunately, there is no "miracle cure" for treating these injuries, but they can be very painful and frustrating so they are worth mentioning.

Usually the result of direct trauma, rib sprains and bruises are the most common chest injuries that I see. They can hurt just as much as rib fractures, so can be difficult to diagnose just based on symptoms, and, like fracture can often make it hurt even to breathe. Sprain and bruises generally heal faster than fractures, but not by much. Even sprains and bruises can take weeks or even months to heal completely. They often make it hurt even to breath. Years ago, we would wrap and tape these injuries, but we have realized that, unfortunately, this does not help much. Icing the area, avoiding recurrent trauma (which is harder than you would think since these areas seem to be magnets for repeat injury), taking NSAIDs, and being patient are your best bet.

If the pain is unusually severe or prolonged, you may wish to consider getting an X-ray to rule out a fracture. Unfortunately, even if a rib is broken, there is not much more than the above treatment that can be done to help with pain control or healing. Thankfully, rib fractures are usually not serious and heal on their own. One exception, however, is in the rare case when the fractured rib actually punctures the lung, resulting in what is called a pneumothorax. This causes in profound, and usually immediate, shortness of breath, and is a true medical emergency.

Back Pain

Back pain is one of the most common complaints seen in almost every doctor's office. It seems to be "part and parcel" of the human condition. Twinges of pain or a pulled or sprained back are not usually cause for great concern, but sometimes the pain is severe and unrelenting. Of course, ice and NSAIDs can help, but severe injuries can take considerable time to heal. If you have been in the martial arts for long, you have likely realized that this can and will happen from time to time.

One of the best things you can do for yourself is to learn how to *prevent* back injuries. In general, being active, participating in the martial arts, strengthening your core muscles and proper stretching can help prevent the most serious injuries. If you have a recurrent problem with back pain, a daily stretching and strengthening regimen is likely indicated. Above and beyond that, you want to learn to lift properly. Bending at the knees, when possible, can help. Below are some exercises and stretches to help prevent back injury:

BACK EXERCISES

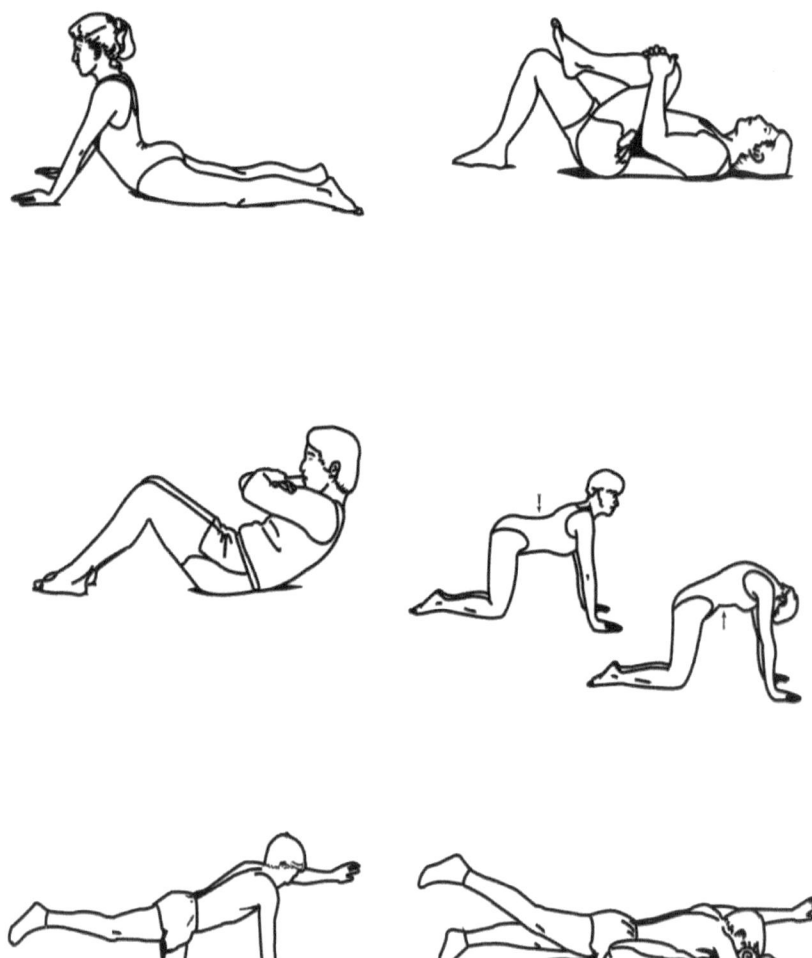

If you are picking up something light-weight, such as a shoe or small ball, you can alleviate the pressure on your back by lifting one leg behind you as you bend down to pick it up. It is still safer to bend at the knees, but if you are tired of squatting down, this is a trick that most golfers know well.

A similar approach can be taken with neck pain. Ice and stretching can be a great way to relieve pain and prevent future injuries. Adding some range of motion exercises such as chin-to-chest, head side-to-side, and head rolls can help prevent future pain or injuries. Care should be taken with back or neck pain that causes shooting pain, numbness, or weakness down the arms or legs. This may mean that you have a spinal cord injury, canal narrowing, or nerve impingement (compression).

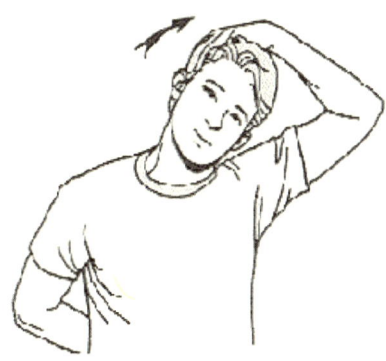

Chapter 12

Injuries to the Head

There are many types of injuries that can occur to the head, almost all of which are potentially serious. I would like to focus here on the prevention and treatment of concussions. Recent media attention has focused on the frequent occurrence of concussions in the sport of football. Recurrent head trauma can result in a condition called chronic traumatic encephalopathy (CTE), or dementia pugilistica as it was originally named. While the media has recently focused on the sport of football when discussing head injuries, this condition was first recognized in boxers. In the early 20th century, the bizarre behavior of prize fighters was referred to being "punch drunk". With recurrent blast injuries to the head CTE has been recognized at autopsy even in amateur football players as young as 17.[2]

Symptoms of CTE include depression, dementia, mood changes, memory loss, and suicidal behavior. Tragically, in 2012, former NFL star Junior Seau took his own life. On autopsy, his brain pathology showed evidence of CTE. It is impossible to say for certain that this was the cause of his suicide, but it is certainly concerning.

One of the most frightening moments for a martial artist, student or instructor, is the knockout. In competition, a knockout is often the goal of your adversary. In daily practice, however, it should be the goal of all involved to avoid it. Some people seem to have the proverbial "chin of steel," meaning that they are able to

---

[2] In 2010, Nathan Styles, a high school football player and Owen Thomas, a college football player, were both posthumously diagnosed with chronic traumatic encephalopathy. They were 17 and 21 years old respectively.

take a beating and keep going. They never seem to get knocked out. While this may seem like a blessing, to a competitive martial artist, it can actually be quite dangerous. Whether you are knocked out or not, even a single well-timed blow can result in some neurologic injury, namely, a concussion.

A concussion, as defined in the medical literature, is often referred to as a mild traumatic brain injury (MTBI). The American Academy of Neurology defines concussion as a "trauma-induced alteration in mental status that may or may not involve loss of consciousness."[3] For years, coaches, athletes, and physicians have been misled into thinking that if they are not knocked out the injury must not be as serious. The majority of concussions do *not* result in any loss of consciousness, and as a result, often go unrecognized.[4] This is unfortunate, as repeated medical studies have demonstrated that even head trauma that does not result in a loss of consciousness can have serious consequences.

Taking it one step further, the trauma does not always have to be directly to the head for there to be neurologic damage. A strong blow to the body can result in transmitted force to the head, resulting in indirect trauma to the brain. Any injury that results in rapid acceleration and/or deceleration of the brain can cause a concussion. Most commonly, this is a direct blow, but not always.

How does a concussion happen? Any violent shock, blow, or jolt to the head can cause the brain to shift inside the skull. The

---

[3] Practice parameter: the management of concussion in sports (summary statement). Report of the Quality Standards Subcommittee. Neurology 1997; 48:581.

[4] Relationship between concussion and neuropsychological performance in college football players. JAMA 1999; 282:964-70.

brain is a soft gelatin-like material floating inside the skull in the cerebrospinal fluid. The hard skull is designed to protect the brain from any direct injury; however, any rapid acceleration or deceleration can result in the brain shifting inside the skull and colliding against the hard bone. This can result in anything from a minor bruise to severe life-threatening injuries.

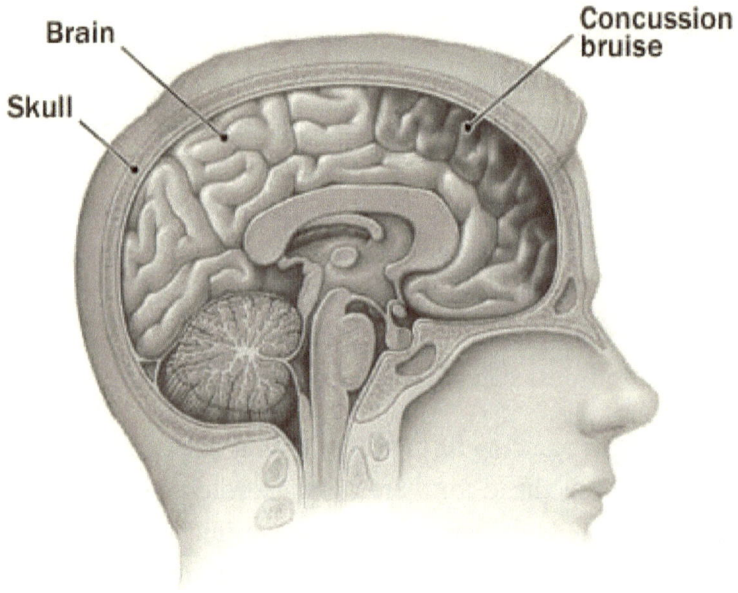

Figure 1: Cross-sectional view of the brain and skull showing a concussion bruise.

So how do you know if you or someone else has sustained a concussion? The first step is to suspect concussion anytime there is trauma to the head. A higher level of suspicion needs to be raised anytime somebody is exhibiting unusual behavior. The most common symptoms are confusion and memory loss - if someone is confused or forgetful following any type of head trauma, a concussion is likely. There are other symptoms to watch for as well. These include nausea or vomiting, ringing in the ears (tinnitus), headache, drowsiness, and dizziness.

It is valuable for the medical professional, and interesting for the martial artist, to understand how and why a knockout or unconsciousness occurs. Alertness and consciousness are maintained and regulated by the reticular activating system (RAS). This is a bundle of nerves that travels through the midbrain and signals the higher levels of brain function (known as executive functions, and including things such as reasoning, planning, and working memory), to continue. If there is rapid or severe enough torsion (twisting force) at the base of the skull, this temporarily disrupts transmission through the reticular activating system. As a result, consciousness is lost. Thus, what would otherwise seem to be milder blows can also result in a loss of consciousness if the appropriate target is struck a specific manner.

Conversely, an individual can sustain a severe, even devastating blow, but not lose consciousness, if the blow does not affect the reticular activating system. Severe blows can lead to bleeding under the skull. However, they may not necessarily affect the reticular activating system until they become sufficiently large that the damage is irreversible. One such frightening injury called an epidural hematoma. Here, bleeding occurs beneath the skull but outside the lining (dura) of the brain. The initial injury is followed by a period of mental clarity lasting a few hours. Then, once the bleeding becomes large enough to shift the brain (and effect the reticular activating system), the patient becomes sleepy and/or confused, eventually losing consciousness and possibly even dying.

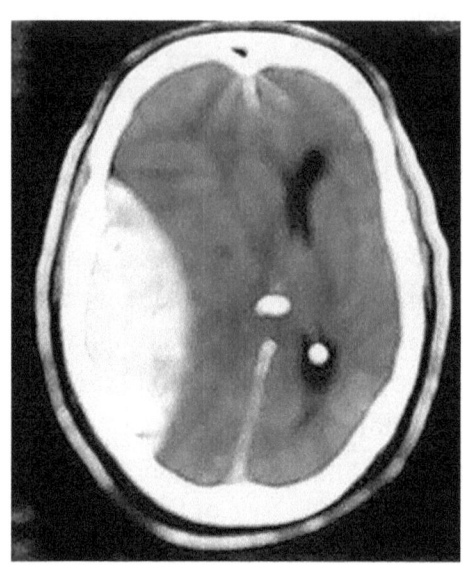

Figure 2: Epidural Hematoma

Consequently, anytime somebody is knocked out it is a good idea for them to be evaluated a medical professional, preferably in an emergency department where radiographic imaging is available. There are too many accounts of "it's just a bump on the head" that have led to disastrous consequence, so whenever there is any doubt it is better to be safe than sorry.

An understanding of this physiology can give a martial artist a better understanding of why some blows result in a loss of consciousness while others do not. It is often said that it is the blow that you don't see coming that causes the greatest amount of damage. This occurs because the person being struck is unable to prepare him or herself for the oncoming blow. As a result, the neck muscles, and the body as a whole, are not prepared to resist or counter-act the force. The resulting blow then has much greater strength, by means of greater acceleration and torsion that the brain then experiences. This makes it more likely to injure the reticular activating system or cause shearing of the brain's blood vessels, resulting in cerebral hemorrhage (bleeding in the brain). This is one of the reasons that the "sucker punch" is so dangerous.

It is invaluable to have martial arts instructors and coaches trained in the basics of a concussion. That way, the symptoms can be recognized early and the appropriate evaluation and intervention can take place immediately. In general, common sense should dictate a return to any vigorous physical activity. The person should be pain and symptom free before any return. If there is a more severe concussion or a repeated concussion an even more cautious approach should be taken.

When in doubt, a medical professional should be consulted. There are recently-updated guidelines regarding the approach to concussions and the timing of a return to activity. The most recent guidelines recommend not returning to activity until the athlete is symptom free. In addition, the return should be gradual. The athlete should be allowed to participate only in non-contact practice before returning to full training. In more severe cases, it may be necessary to seek out a neurologist or a physician who has significant knowledge and experience with concussion diagnosis and treatment in order to determine the best course of action.

The best way to prevent a concussion is to use common sense. First, practice safely. This means to wear appropriate protective gear. In the martial arts, this includes protective headgear, protective gloves, and a mouthpiece. In addition, always practice under supervision of a trained coach or instructor. It is also important to remember that practice is exactly that, practice. It is not a real competition, let alone a real fight. It is a learning opportunity. You are not there to be hurt or to hurt others. You are there to train, and to learn. Professional athletes get paid millions of dollars to put their bodies (and brains) on the line. For most of us who participate in the martial arts recreationally, it is not necessary (or wise) to do the same.

For those of you who are professional or semi-professional athletes it is important that you undergo a medical evaluation and have a professional coach and trainer. Otherwise, you are taking an unnecessary risk. I would also say that even for those of you who compete in martial arts at the highest levels, think of the number of training sessions that you must go through before a single competitive event. Often times you spend tens, if not hundreds, of hours preparing for a single competition. If you sustain concussions during training, you are increasing your risk of permanent damage a hundred-fold. For all athletes, at all levels, train smart!

Let's review a few of the important points about a concussion:

- A concussion is a mild brain injury due to trauma.
- It is typically due to a high-velocity impact that may or may not result in a loss of consciousness (a knockout).
- A concussion is typically characterized, by confusion, loss of memory, difficulty focusing, nausea, or headache.
- It is important that martial arts coaches and instructors recognize a concussion early and keep the martial artist safe and away from contact or competition until the symptoms completely resolve.

- If the symptoms last more than 15 minutes, if there is a loss of consciousness, or if there is any doubt at all as to the severity of the injury, a medical evaluation should be performed.

It is important to remember that it is not necessary for someone to lose consciousness, in order for them to sustain a concussion. Also, multiple concussions that occur in a short period of time can result in serious and permanent brain damage. Second impact syndrome (SIS) occurs when there are recurrent brain injuries in a short period of time. This can lead to permanent neurological injury and even death. While this condition is not common, young athletes appear to be more prone to SIS.

If there is any doubt that someone has suffered a concussion, they should be evaluated. Do not let them return to play, no matter how much they insist, until they are fully and completely recovered, and if necessary cleared, by a medical professional. If the martial artist does not seem to be acting quite like him or herself, there is a good chance that he or she has sustained a concussion.

I would like to conclude by emphasizing the importance of prevention. Do all that you can to prevent concussions in yourself, your training partners, and in your students. Contact training, such as sparring, should only be conducted in a controlled, supervised setting. The appropriate protective gear should always be worn. If there is an injury, stop and evaluate - do not push through and risk further harm to yourself or others. You will find that by doing this, not only can you still train hard, you can actually train harder, by avoiding unnecessary injuries. As I said before, above all else, train *smart*!

Section III – Optimizing Performance

Chapter 13

Competition Preparation –

This section is taken from a handout that I created specifically for students who are preparing for their black belt test. It is a grueling test and over the years there have been numerous injuries, ranging from very minor to very severe, most of which could have been avoided with proper preparation. The advice I give below is readily adaptable to fit almost any competitive sporting or athletic environment. Simply substitute your event for the test described below as you read.

You have come a long way in preparing for your black belt, and for that you are to be congratulated. You have put years into studying karate and memorizing the basics, sets, forms, and techniques that are required to earn your black belt. You will need more than that, though, if you want to be successful on the days of the test. You will need to be mentally tough as well as physically ready. In order to make the test as safe as possible, I would like to make a few recommendations.

First, you need to understand how tough the test really is. Most of those stories you have heard from the older black belts are true. The test is not easy. No two tests are exactly the same, but they are all quite rigorous. You need to mentally prepare yourself for this fact well ahead of time and accept it. Your test will not be different. It will be hard.

We are going to do our best to make the test as safe for you as possible. In order for that to happen, though, you need to be prepared. That doesn't just mean memorizing your curriculum. You need to physically prepare yourself for this event like it is a major undertaking, because it is.

You would not run a marathon or climb Mount Everest without preparing yourself. Just knowing how to run or how to climb will not get you to the finish line or to the top of the mountain. Similarly, just knowing your techniques will not get you through a black belt test.

So, if you are considering testing, how do you prepare? Beyond knowing your testing requirements, you need to make sure that you are physically healthy enough for the test. If you have not seen a doctor and had an exam in more than 2 years, I would strongly urge you to go. For those over 30, a physical exam should be done every 1-2 years. For men over the age of 45, and women over 55, you will want to make sure your physician understands the rigorous test you are about to undergo and ensures that your heart is healthy enough for the test.

Once you have been cleared by your physician, you need to accept responsibility for preparing yourself for the test. You and you alone will get yourself ready for and through this test. Your instructors, coaches, and classmates will teach you, guide you, and support you, but ultimately you are the one responsible for preparing yourself for this test. Just *being* in class is not enough. Wearing the black belt means that you did more than just show up. You have to give it everything you've got and you can't do that if you're not ready.

Understand what the test involves so that you can prepare for it. While every test is a little bit different, the requirements and the structure generally remain the same. The test is currently run over two days with the first day being the fitness test and the second day being your curriculum test. If you have not witnessed the fitness test before, you should make it a point to do so well before your own test day. You will typically get the chance to do a trial run of the fitness test two weeks prior, which you absolutely *should not miss*. You should, however, be ready long before the pretest. The fitness test typically involves a three mile run, followed by pull-ups, push-ups, sit-ups, 1000 strikes, 500 kicks, and sprints.

The curriculum test will be similar to your brown belt test, but harder! You will need to be ready to perform ALL of the basics, forms, sets, and techniques (in the air and on a body) at a black belt level. You will then need to spar up to 10 (or more) rounds at anywhere from light to full contact. You need to be ready to fight at all ranges against various opponents that will be better rested and bigger than you are. You should take full advantage of the boxing, Muay Thai, and Jiu Jitsu classes available at the gym. It will improve your conditioning and help you get ready for the sparring portion of your black belt test.

Let's get down to the details of what I would recommend you do to get ready for the test. This is similar advice to what I would give a patient who is running a marathon.

Water is your friend! You should drink plenty of water in the days and weeks leading up to the test. I would consider 64 ounces to be the absolute minimum that you need while training. On hard training days you will likely need twice that amount. Don't wait until the day of the test to hydrate. During vigorous exercise the stomach does not absorb fluids as well, so you need to drink, but not too much! To avoid dehydration on the day(s) of the test you should be getting plenty of water well ahead of time.

Eat a healthy, balanced diet. Use common sense here. You do need carbohydrates as a source of energy, but if you don't normally eat pasta, a huge plate of spaghetti before the test is going to end up in the bushes (just ask some of the black belts!). Also, if you are overweight, you will almost certainly lose weight in training for your black belt exam, but now is NOT the time to starve yourself. You need a healthy diet so that your body keeps working and your muscles don't cramp up in the middle of the test.

Don't forget electrolytes. For a typical class or workout water is enough. For the test days and on your hard training days you may want to consider a sports drink with electrolytes. When we exercise vigorously for over 2 hours our body needs sugar, salt, and other electrolytes to operate at its highest capacity. If you don't normally drink Gatorade, or similar fluids, test day is not the time to find out how it works for you. I would recommend trying it on your hard training days and incorporating it come test day if it works for you.

Get yourself ready for the hot weather! As you know, the black belt test happens every year during the summer, and Poway is not known for its cool July weather. The average high temperature in July is 90 degrees and you need to be prepared! Because of this, you need to be extra careful to make sure that you drink enough fluids. You should also get yourself acclimated to training in the heat. You are going to need to get yourself out of the air conditioning and run and train outside.

Above all else, prepare for test day by training like every day is test day. In the months and weeks leading up to the test you should be running, sparring, kicking, punching, and doing pull-ups, push-ups, and sit-ups. This is in addition to your curriculum review that you are doing in class. Only *you* can get yourself ready for this test. Just showing up to class will not be enough. If you follow my advice, though, and train like you mean it, you will succeed. It will be the test of a lifetime. You will wear your belt proudly and tell all the new black belt candidates about how hard your test really was! In the meantime, go get ready!

Conclusion

As a martial athlete you are on a rigorous journey to a better and stronger you. There will be bumps and bruises along the way. Some will be minor and others will make you want to give up and quit. Understanding your body will help you to grow throughout the journey. Take your time and realize that there is no rush to get anywhere. It is much more about the journey than the destination.

As part of this journey you will learn a lot about yourself and grow mentally and physically. Skills will be gained that may one day save your life. An important part of the journey is to listen to your body, as well as to your instructor. This will help you to know when to slow down, when to push harder, or when to take a rest.

Above all else, train smart and don't give up. The tips in this book will help you better prepare for, and get the most out of, your training. Though injuries inevitably happen, you can prevent many, if not most of them. Once you *are* injured, however, an understanding how your body works can help you to treat the injuries properly and to heal faster and more-completely.

Bonus Section: Kenpo and the Rule of Threes

PREFACE

I remember the saying as "Great things come in pairs," but apparently Grandmaster Edmund Parker Sr. did not agree. Modern American Kenpo Karate is riddled with a cacophony of tertiary references. This is not really inappropriate or accidental. The triangle has been around for longer than modern society. We have the beloved triangle musical instrument, which I perfected in the first grade Christmas pageant, the triangle choke of jiu-jitsu, which I have yet to perfect, and the various triangles of geometry including, equilateral, Isosceles, and scalene. The triangle is present in architecture, art, and religious imagery. Most notable is the Star of David[i] which is essentially a double triangle and I would be remiss not to mention the concept of the Trinity which dominates modern Christian thinking and ideology.

INTRODUCTION

The triangle is the dominant shape and symbol on the American Kenpo Alliance patch. It is a structure that conveys power, suggests beauty, and in the properly trained hands of a Kenpo practitioner, is positively lethal. The idea of splitting your opponents, getting off the line, and attacking your opponent's weak side can all be better explained and understood by studying the triangle. It could be argued that once the student understands the line and the circle, the triangle is the next step. This would be true both in primary education and in understanding the universal pattern.

The universal pattern is formed by drawing a circle first. This is then split into eight slices by drawing four intersecting lines. A square is then drawn in the middle that connects these endpoints. This creates a total of 22 separate triangles. The ends of the all eight lines are then connected and four circles are added completing the two-dimensional universal pattern. This can then be expanded into a three-dimensional version which by extrapolation contains an infinite number of triangles.[ii]

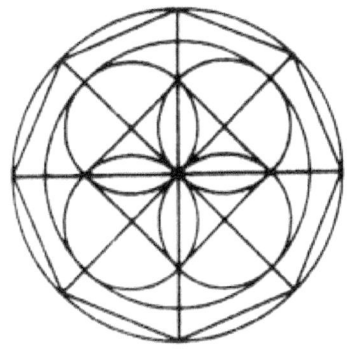

Fig. 1 – Universal Pattern

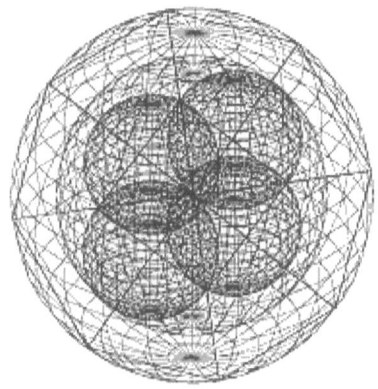

Fig. 2 – Three-dimensional Universal Pattern

OVERVIEW

What I am primarily interested in, though, is the multiplicity of triplets, rules of three, three phases, three stages, and the three divisions that exist within Kenpo. Please consider the following for a moment:

The Three Divisions of the Art:

1. Basics (including forms and sets)
2. Self-defense
3. Freestyle

The Three Phase Concept:

1. Ideal Phase
2. What if Phase
3. Formulation Phase

The Three Stages of Learning:

1. Primitive Stage
2. Mechanical Stage
3. Spontaneous Stage

The Three States of Motion:

1. Solid
2. Liquid
3. Gas

The Three Viewpoints:

1. My viewpoint
2. Opponent's viewpoint

3. Bystander's viewpoint

Analogy of Writing:

1. Print
2. Script
3. Shorthand

Analogy of Language:

1. Letters
2. Words
3. Sentences

Analogy of References:

1. Appendix
2. Dictionary
3. Encyclopedia:

Dimensional Zone Theory:

1. Height Zones
2. Width Zones
3. Depth Zones

In addition, while there are four stages of range there is a subdivision which is the three stages of contact. The first stage of range is out of contact while the remaining three ranges are:

1. Within Contact
2. Contact Penetration
3. Contact Manipulation

For purposes of comparison, the three stages of sport fighting, from a mixed martial arts perspective:

1. Stand up
2. Clinch
3. Ground fighting

Consider further the tree divisions of a human being from a philosophical standpoint:

1. Body
2. Mind
3. Spirit

Those interested in a discussion of these three divisions can look forward to the upcoming work of my instructor, Master Barry Barker.

Of course, even more examples exist and more could be discovered or invented. It is not my purpose to catalogue every possible grouping of three that exists in Kenpo. Rather, it is my intention to prevail upon the reader the numerous cases of its existence. There is a rule of threes in writing that placing sayings and ideas into groupings of threes is inherently more effective, more memorable and more persuasive. Whether or not that is the case, it is clear that Mr. Parker, consciously or not, included many groupings of three in his Kenpo terminology. Further, I would like to explore how these groupings relate to each other, differ from each other, and how they can be used to improve our understanding of Kenpo, martial arts and motion in general.

There is a tremendous amount of crossover between some of these categories. While all of these categories have value and use in understanding and teaching the art, I intend to focus primarily on the three divisions, the three phases, the three stages of learning and the three states of motion. Some time will be spent on the others but these four provide so much of the foundation of our understanding of the art. A deeper understanding of these categories and how they relate will help propel both the student and the teacher along their Kenpo journey.

THE THREE DIVISIONS OF THE ART

Let us review for a moment the three divisions of the art. The first division is the basics. Interestingly, Mr. Parker chose to include the sets and forms in the basics when discussing his three divisions.[iii] This was in direct contrast to his Japanese predecessors and contemporaries who split Karate-do into Kihon (basics), Kata (forms) and Kumite (sparring). Mr. Parker's emphasis on self-defense and self-defense techniques has led many to consider them the heart of the art. This was distinctly different from traditional 20th century and onward Karate-do where the self-defense applications where considered hidden moves, applications, or waza which were for the more advanced students to understand, discover and study. Beginning students were not typically introduced directly to combat and self-defense scenarios until later in their training under the traditional Japanese methodology. While there are certainly those who approach their training similarly the omission of self-defense from the traditional Karate-do, and Mr. Parker's direct inclusion of the same in his art was not accidental.

Similar to the Japanese, though, he felt basics were of primary importance, hence they were listed first. Originally, the sets were seen as a collection of basics upon which to build the art. The original forms, emphasized basics put together in a sequence. It was the later forms that emphasized the self-defense techniques, but that was not the case in the earliest forms of Kenpo Karate.[iv]

Moving on to the third division of the art, it is important to note another distinction here between Mr. Parker's terminology and that of traditional Karate-do.[v] Traditional Karate-do speaks of kumite or sparring as the third division of the art. Mr. Parker, on the other hand, considered the third division of the art to be freestyle. On their faces these would seem to be very similar concepts. The Japanese word kumite however specifically excludes actual fighting or even competition sparring as there are other specific words for that. Randori, for example connotes competition based sparring. Mr. Parker on the other hand intended for freestyle to be an all-inclusive term that included both competition and street freestyle.[vi]

THE IMPORTANCE OF FREESTYLE

In Kenpo today we do not use the word freestyle as much as it was once used. It was a popular term in the 1970s and 1980s to describe the sparring or fighting divisions in tournaments. This eventually became associated with foam-dipped sparring gear and "tap fighting" and the word has fallen out of common use at least in the local martial arts training centers today. Understanding, how Mr. Parker used and intended the word can heighten our understanding of the art.

Street freestyle is the spontaneous expression of Kenpo in the street, where it is intended to be used. Street freestyle is the ultimate expression of Kenpo. Mr. Parker never explicitly stated this, but for the careful reader it is implied in his writings. Further, in conversations with some of the personal students and first generation Kenpo Black Belts this has been repeatedly confirmed.[vii] With that said, all three divisions of the art are required for the appropriate development of the student. In the words of Grandmaster Ed Parker:

> With self-defense assuming much and freestyle basically assuming no injury has been rendered, one might question the value of both methods of training. Both methods are essential, providing the student is made aware of their

ultimate purpose. When faced with a crisis, the training you have acquired in both areas will merge and its value will become apparent. For you will discover that the knowledge you obtain from freestyle training will have taught you maneuverability, to increase you reflexes, strike with speed, maintain proper distance, increase your accuracy, etc. Then when injury does occur to your opponent, rendering him helpless, extemporaneous movements that stem from self-defense training can be utilized at random. When this occurs, every opportunity to use other techniques can be taken advantage of. At this very instant, the marriage of self-defense and freestyle knowledge begin to produce positive results that lead to an assured victory.[viii]

Clearly all three divisions of the art are essential. Basics lay the foundation, self-defense techniques teach the movements, and freestyle teaches the spontaneous application. All three must be present in training or else you will only succeed in becoming a partial artist.

TRAINNG METHODS BASED ON THE RULE OF THREES

At Poway Martial Arts and as members of the American Kenpo Alliance we are taught a comprehensive freestyle (or sparring) curriculum. It includes basic sparring, boxing, kickboxing, Muay Thai, wrestling, judo, jiu-jitsu, and mixed martial arts techniques in the curriculum. In addition, we have access to incredible instructors and coaches who specialize in most, if not all of these areas. In order to maximize your growth as a martial artist appropriate time and attention to these areas must be applied. With that said, ultimate expression of your Kenpo will also depend on an understanding of the art itself. Without appropriate basics and self-defense techniques, along with an understanding of the architecture of the system and how to teach it you stand the risk of becoming a jack of all trades but a master of none.

Freestyle and sparring should not be relegated completely to the sport realm, however. If that is the only time that one practices freestyle there will be a noticeable gap between one's self-defense knowledge and his or hers ability to extemporaneously apply it in the street. Drills can and should be developed to bridge the gap between the two. How often have you noticed that sparring looks nothing like Kenpo? How often have you noticed that attackers do not attack realistically? And even if they do, they offer little or no resistance, standing there like a statue while someone dances around them doing a 17 move extension.

We need to be able to bridge the gap between self-defense and freestyle. Our techniques need to be trained realistically. We need to have realistic attacks. We need to understand the nature, the context, and the intent behind the attacks. When we attack we should be certain that the defender will know it if they do not defend realistically. Otherwise, we are wasting our time. Further there needs to be appropriate responses from the attacker. They need to respond to the eye and groin strikes as they actually have been hit. On the body strikes we actually should hit! What that also means is that if we don't control or strike accordingly that the attacker is to respond as he would in the street, not just stand there! Of course, at a very beginner level when the student is learning the technique a compliant posture should be assumed so that the student can be coached through the appropriate movements in a safe and effective manner. However, once the techniques have been learned, especially at the upper belt levels there should be significant contact and resistance applied.

At the next level we need to begin to introduce spontaneity into the equation of our self-defense formula. The three stages of learning are primitive, mechanical and spontaneous. When the student learns the technique it is primitive and the attacker is compliant. At an intermediate level the defender is mechanical, with contact, and the defender offers modest resistance. At an advanced level not only should the attacker offer sufficient resistance there should also be a level of spontaneity to the attack itself. For safety, this should be introduced in stages with appropriate safety equipment. At first the roles of attacker and defender should be defined. The attack itself should be defined. The attackers and defenders may change roles and take turns attacking each other. Moderate resistance and contact should be strongly encouraged once a basic familiarity with the techniques is assumed.

At the next level we expand the attacks into a broader category. The attacks can be based on type such as is used in the web of knowledge. You can progress from grabs and tackles, pushes, punches, kicks, hugs and holds, locks and chokes, weapons, multiple attackers, and combination attacks. As the skill level and confidence of the students increases the attacks can become completely random. The technique choice for the response will be left to the student. It may be a single self-defense technique, a sparring technique, a combination or something completely original.

The next phase, which is the most dangerous, is to have the attackers and defenders spontaneously reverse roles. With sufficient skill this becomes a constant exchange where the attacker is also defending and vice-versa. This essentially becomes sparring or uninhibited freestyle. The hope is with appropriate training and introduction that bad habits ingrained by traditional point sparring can be eradicated while maintaining the lessons of spontaneity, range and timing while maintaining the safety of all involved. This has been done in various arts other than Kenpo with consistent success. It is not dissimilar from the training methods found in sports, law enforcement, or medicine. I have personally conducted classes with this method and have had consistently good results. What tends to happen in already skilled martial artists is that the learning curve is flattened, confidence increases, and the applicability of already held skills becomes readily apparent.

THE THREE PHASE CONCEPT

Returning to the concept of the rule of threes and Kenpo many similarities can be drawn from the examples above in the three divisions of the art. As basics, self-defense, and freestyle are learned and applied the student will naturally move through the three stages of learning: primitive, mechanical and spontaneous. This will be much more readily apparent with more advance students. Those just beginning will need to spend a much greater portion of their time on basics in order to assure that degradation of skill does not occur as pressure, stress, and random attacks are forced upon them.

The three phase concept is readily applicable as well. The students are able to explore the what if phase. With the assistance of their instructors, while reinforcing proper basics, an appropriate formulation phase can be reached. This is best reserved for more advanced students and instructors. For beginning students it will tend to lead to improper formulations and limiting of their own skills and horizons as they will inevitably gravitate to specific built-in tendencies. This must be avoided by forcing them to learn the new skills and techniques and then only formulate they own when they have sufficient understanding of the art and guidance from their instructor. Instructors must be careful as they use the three phase concept to develop new or improve existing techniques for their students. Care must be taken not to discard old information by deeming it non-functional until it is appropriately understood. New or updated techniques should be sufficiently evaluated and tested before they are included in the curriculum.

THE THREE STATES OF MOTION

As you watch your students grow you will notice them moving through the three states of motion. These bear many resemblances to the three stages of motion with fine differences. Solid motion and primitive motion are quite similar. Good solid motion can also be fairly mechanical. That is not a bad thing, but a sign of progress. When the solid motions become liquid it begins to move past the mechanical stage, though it does not become completely spontaneous until it enters the gaseous state. Liquid motion does have a certain level of spontaneity just as liquid will fill a container to a certain level. However, gaseous motion completely, automatically, and spontaneously fills its space. So while there are similarities between the states of motion and the stages of learning there are differences as well. Being able to achieve effective and spontaneous movement should be a goal for all students. Once this is achieved, if it is effectively practiced and refined, a gaseous state of motion can be achieved.

THE THREE STAGES OF CONTACT

We discussed above progressive training, using all three divisions of the art which culminates in freestyle training. The three stages of contact, namely in contact, contact penetration and contact manipulation will be automatically ingrained into the student in a way that would not be possible with self-defense or freestyle training alone. The transition will be seamless from one stage to another as the student learns to blend what he has learned into an automatic response to a given stimuli. The same is true for the three stages of MMA sport fighting. Your students will learn to attack and defend while standing, in the clinch, and on the ground. This will be part of the natural progression as they work their way through the various categories of attacks from the web of knowledge. Certain efforts should be made to avoid a specific sport-fighting mentality. While this has its place, a certain emphasis should be placed on the nature of Kenpo, what we are training for, and the ultimate goal of combat efficacy, and both competence and excellence at street freestyle.

PUTTING IT ALL TOGETHER

Now would be a good time to review the attached appendix if you have not already. First, you will see the three divisions of the art: basics, self-defense and freestyle. This is the order in which the Kenpo system should be taught. As appropriate self-defense techniques are modified, updated, or added the three phase concept becomes for the instructor and the most advanced students. Using the training methods discussed above, along with a foundational understanding of Kenpo and street self-defense, the three phase concept can be used to maximize the efficacy of the self-defense techniques. As the instructor teaches these techniques to the student he will see them move through the three stages of learning: primitive, mechanical, and spontaneous. The spontaneous stage can be developed and tested by incorporating random attacks, stress training, and controlled freestyle into the training curriculum. As the overall student develops we will see them develop higher levels or states of motion. The three states of motion are: solid, liquid and gas.

In conclusion, understanding the terminology of Kenpo will bring the martial artist to an understanding of the numerous places where groups of three occur. Deeper understanding of the three divisions of the art, the three phase concept, the three stages of learning, and the three states of motion will deepen your understanding of Kenpo. This in turn, will better enable you to understand, dissect, explain, and teach the art of Kenpo. After all, it is our goal to reach combat efficacy, and to teach valid and functional self-defense. Without that we simply become what Mr. Parker referred to as a "salesman of motion". A salesman of motion can explain the art, talk it up, impress his internet followers, and perhaps even recruit a successful commercial following. However, he has not internalized the art and is not capable of spontaneous movement. As such, he has not yet graduated into becoming a mechanic of motion who can dissect, put back together, and apply what he has been taught. Mr. Parker actually had a third category (surprise!) which we should all strive for – that is to become an engineer of motion. An engineer of motion not only understands the motion that already exists and that has been given to him, but he is also capable of designing, improving and understanding motion to such a level that it becomes movement. He is both the composer and the director of the symphony. He becomes the creator and the teacher. The salesman can talk the talk, while the mechanic can walk the walk, but the engineer transcends these and truly creates. The differences to the casual observer and to the untrained eye and mind may be subtle, but to the sophisticated practitioner and the dedicated student the difference is both obvious and of tremendous importance.

AFTERWORD

While I continue on my own path to become an engineer of motion, my hope is that for those who read and truly study some of my simple thoughts and the writings and teachings of Grandmaster Ed Parker, that they may be accelerated along on their own journey. Thank you for reading.

APPENDIX

The following is designed to help the student and reader better visualize, remember, and distinguish the similarities and differences between the most commonly discussed divisions of three in Kenpo. There is a strong common thread that is not accidental. However, care must be taken not to blur the lines and forget the distinctions between the various subcategories. Basics, for example, can be primitive, spontaneous or mechanical. Freestyle can be solid, liquid or gas. Of course, as one better understands these divisions it will enhance his understanding of Kenpo and improve your ability to teach others and help them on their own journey.

3 DIVISIONS	3 PHASES	3 STAGES	3 STATES OF MOTION
1. Basics	Ideal	Primitive	Solid
2. Self-Defense	What If	Mechanical	Liquid
3. Freestyle	Formulation	Spontaneous	Gas

[i] The Star of David of Shield of David is the symbol most commonly associated with the State of Israel and the Jewish religion. It is essentially two triangles with one rotated 180 degrees and superimposed on the other.

[ii] Parker, Ed. *Ed Parker's Kenpo Karate: Sophisticated Basics Volume 1*. The first part of a planned video series by Master Parker. Unfortunately only two volumes were ever completed and released.

[iii] Parker, Ed. *Infinite Insights into Kenpo. Volume 1*. Delsby Publications. 1982: 43-53.

[iv] In discussions with various Kenpo seniors it has become apparent that the original Kenpo forms were Short 1 through Short 3. While Short 3 is considered the first of the encyclopedia forms (as opposed to a dictionary form) it is somewhat of an abbreviated encyclopedia by comparison. Long 3 through Form 6 came later with Form 7 and Form 8 coming much later still.

[v] It should be noted that the author does not intend to disparage Japanese Karate. Quite to the contrary, the traditional arts when properly trained can be tremendously beneficial. The author has trained in both Wado-ryu and Shotokan and the apparent differences in terminology are interesting primarily to see how Mr. Parker framed, designed, and intended the art to be taught and understood.

[vi] Parker, Ed. *Infinite Insights into Kenpo. Volume 1*. Delsby Publications. 1982: 43-53.

[vii] Personal conversation between the author and Mr. Dennis Conatser, Sr. Scottsdale, Arizona. 2007.

[viii] Parker, Ed. *Infinite Insights into Kenpo. Volume 1*. Delsby Publications. 1982: 52-53.